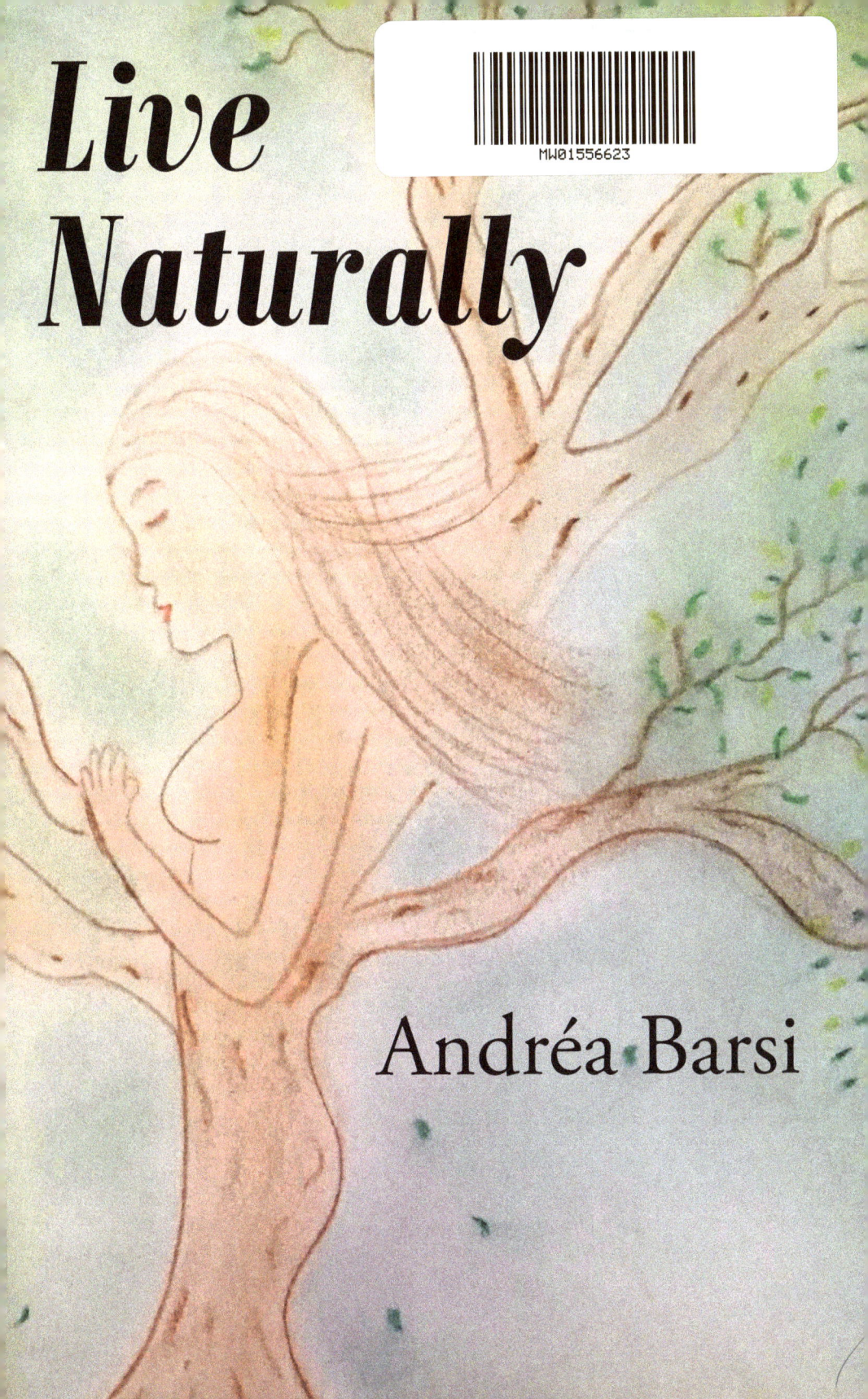

ISBN 978-1-64258-196-6 (paperback)
ISBN 978-1-64258-197-3 (digital)

Copyright © 2018 by Andréa Barsi

All rights reserved. No part of this publication may be reproduced, distributed, or transmitted in any form or by any means, including photocopying, recording, or other electronic or mechanical methods without the prior written permission of the publisher. For permission requests, solicit the publisher via the address below.

Christian Faith Publishing, Inc.
832 Park Avenue
Meadville, PA 16335
www.christianfaithpublishing.com

Printed in the United States of America

Contents

Introduction 7
Chapter 1: Where We Began 9
Chapter 2: Where We Were 20
Chapter 3: My Theories 30
Chapter 4: My Recipes 34
Chapter 5: Breakfast 36
Chapter 6: Soups 56
Chapter 7: Salads 67
Chapter 8: Sides 83
Chapter 9: Sandwiches 99
Chapter 10: Meals 113
Chapter 11: Condiments 132
Chapter 12: Party Time 146
Chapter 13: Desserts 159
Chapter 14: Cravings 180
Chapter 15: Home Remedies 180
Chapter 16: Knowledge Is Power 184
Chapter 17: Water 188
Chapter 18: Apple Cider Vinegar 192
Chapter 19: Kefir 196
Chapter 20: Headaches 199
Chapter 21: Fevers 204
Chapter 22: What About Our Girl 209
Chapter 23: Where Are We Going 219

A lot of what I have written about is the way I have lived and raised my family, the problems since the concussion is remembering and processing and the ability to account for why I do the things I do. I am not looking for acceptance or pity in dealing with the injury I have, but I am looking to help people. Not only the people that may have suffered the same injuries as I have but also the people at a loss of how to get to a whole body wellness. Understanding the ways to nourish and protect your body—the mind, body, and soul are all things we have but do we understand how to have them work in unison? I am not a writer, I just know what works for me and would like to share what I have learned throughout my lifetime and share it with you. I see this as a beginner guide, you will not feel like you are trying anything crazy just starting to adapt to a healthier way of living.

Introduction

I started this project with the thought of having everything in one place, a hope that in the future my daughter will have all of my most precious recipes and home remedies that we share as a family. I realize now that this has probably been a work in progress for years.

When I was in college, I would collect recipes. I have a huge three-ring binder filled, most I have never made, some I have but have completely altered the recipe to the types of ingredients I use. I went to college for business administration and accounting, but had a love for cooking and took extra business classes in the field. In one class I did come up with a plan to opening my own restaurant and had to make a menu for my kitchen. Why do I still hold on to them, who knows, maybe a reminder that I have always been into nutrition and creating ideas to share with family and friends. Or maybe to remind myself of the little dreams I had, as I started out on my own.

Years later, I bought a blank cookbook when my daughter was very small and started writing down my favorite recipes. But throughout the years I have altered the recipes so there are notes all over them or papers hanging out of it that haven't been added yet. I am awful at following recipes as it is, so my meals are always on the fly with the healthiest ingredients available.

As I sit here trying to get all of my thoughts together, I realize I have probably six notebooks with random thoughts, recipes, or ideas written in them. I think it is a good time to finally acknowledge a few things and be okay in speaking about them.

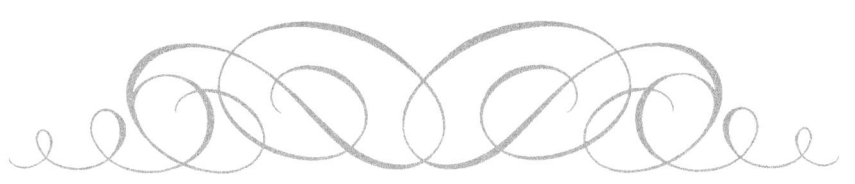

Where We Began

"For I know the plans I have for you,"
declares the Lord, "plans to prosper you
and not to harm you,
plans to give you hope and a future."

—Jeremiah 29:11

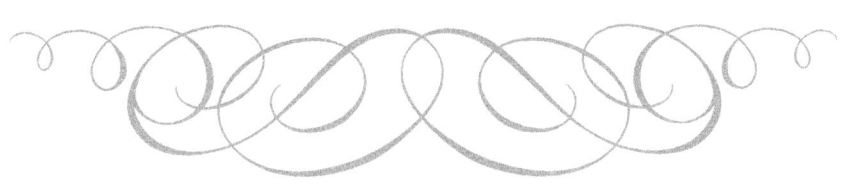

I've been an organic momma even before I was a momma. Have I been perfect? No, no one is perfect, only the creator above. Have I made mistakes? Yes, of course I have, and I'm still learning every day!

I was a teenager during the fat-free generation and like many others at that time, I believed if it was fat-free it had to be amazing for you—all the guilty pleasures with none of the guilt, with no thought whatsoever of what the so called fat-free food was made of. And compared to other food, it was inexpensive, so we were saving money—a no-brainer, right? A meal my boyfriend and I would make often was a grilled cheese masterpiece, a loaf of bakery white Italian bread cut in very thick slices then cut in half and hollowed out. Stuffed with fat-free mozzarella cheese, dipped in fat-free eggs that came in a box. Once fried in a pan with non-fat cooking spray, we would dip these sandwiches in jarred tomato sauce. And for dessert, Snackwell's fat-free cookies of course! I cannot believe this is what we ate, oh, but we did. When I think now of how many chemicals, additives, and sugars would have been in that meal, it floors me we weren't sick all of the time. But back then the stomachaches or bloating would not have made me think they were from what I was eating. Plus, when you are young, your body is very resilient, it can bounce back faster from injuries you may cause by eating certain foods.

My mind-set back then was not what it is today. I did get better in my twenties, I did come to realize the fat-free artificial lifestyle was not a good thing. But I still wanted and thought fat was bad and stayed away from it. So I would eat salads plain, never any dressings, never any cheeses, never any nuts or seeds, and barely any meats. You may be thinking then, what in the world did you eat? Which is a great question, tons of raw and steamed vegetables, organic of course. Lots of plain salads, some chicken, but I am very picky, it has to be overcooked for me to eat it. And my guilty pleasure has always been pizza, when you're from New York, I think that is a given!

LIVE NATURALLY

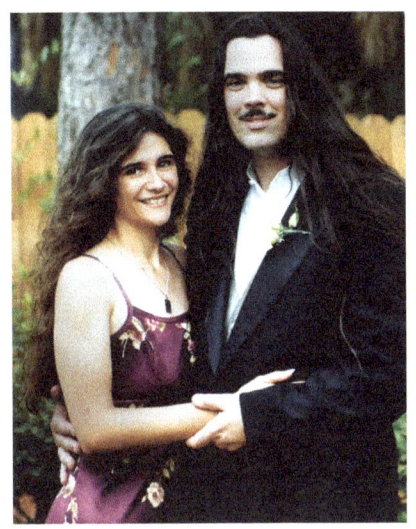

Toward the end of my twenties, I thought I was at my healthiest. I actually was happy with my weight, a feat for most women. I am only 5'3" so 106 being a bit athletic, playing second base in a mixed softball league, rollerblading daily, and working out seemed perfect. But if you asked me back then I would beg to differ.

To find out you're pregnant, what an amazing feeling, I felt so blessed! But the following day to be hemorrhaging and fearful that my happiness would be cut short, not knowing if I did it to myself. I didn't find out I was pregnant till the end of November, beginning of December. I had been sick for weeks and since it was the season of everyone getting the flu, I thought that's what it was. While bowling in our league one Wednesday, my friend said, "Are you sure you're not pregnant?" Of course not, we had been together seven years at this time and my mother had trouble conceiving so I guess I thought I would too. The things we tell ourselves. But yes, I was pregnant and ecstatic so hemorrhaging and a fear of losing my baby was not in the plan and was not going to be what was going on. I was at work and was getting ready to go to lunch, I panicked and called my dad, and he picked me up and took me to my doctors. The office wasn't really interested in what was going on, if you were miscarrying there wasn't much they could do, but I wasn't taking no for an answer and they put me in a room for testing. I never got the whole story, the nurse said I could have lost a twin but since they heard a heartbeat they weren't going to do further tests. That is something I will find out in the afterlife but something I do think about.

Another thing the same nurse told me was I was stage four cancer. *What?* I am twenty-six! I am healthy! I do not feel sick, well, I do, but I assumed it was because I was pregnant. Immediately I was put on bed rest and put through many tests and biopsies. Never did my doctors talk to me about what was going on with my body, we only talked about the baby. I look back now and am so grateful that diagnosis came when I was pregnant because they could not treat me for it. You probably think I am crazy, but I am a person that does not take medication, not even cough medicine, I do all-natural home remedies and have had some reactions to even the simplest of vitamins. I do believe that if I were treated for cancer back then I would not be here today. My daughter is a blessing my Lord has given me and he does everything for a reason. She was meant to be here and I was meant to be her momma.

It made me really sit back and think about what I fed my body inside and out, and how I was going to raise my family in the years to come. At that point I chose to believe I was healthy and carrying a healthy baby. If I was sick I told myself that that meant my baby was healthy and feeling good. Because this was my first and only pregnancy, I didn't have anything to compare it to and I was not going to have that story. I was so happy to become a mother that there was no other outcome—I was going to be a momma and watch my baby grow. Back then I knew nothing about cancer and I had never heard of cervical cancer. I couldn't wrap my mind around that I had it so I put it completely out of my mind and refused to think about it. I didn't question procedures and they wouldn't tell me anyways, the doctors took the place of not upsetting and only telling the positives, how big the baby was, and how her heart rate was, the normal, nothing more. I'm truly glad for that because then, on bed rest, I only watched and read things on babies and parenting. I blessed myself daily with water from Fátima and prayed a lot!

I wish I knew then what I know now about food. I was mostly vegetarian, which was good, but my pregnancy cravings were plain bagels, plain pancakes, and ice cream or frozen yogurt. I had my baby in July so the ice cream craving came on late in my pregnancy and I would only allow myself to have it if we took our evening walk to the ice cream store. We lived about eight to ten blocks away so this was a nice walk for a little treat. Oh, and I can't forget eggplant parmesan sandwiches the last week of my pregnancy during the Italian festival at the foot of my street, I would walk the festival but every night would still come back to the eggplant parmesan and they would make it a sandwich for me. I always thought the bagels and pancakes were more the baby's cravings, as those are my daughter's favorites now. But now after reading so much on cancer and knowing that the body craves those types of carbs and sugars, I shouldn't have given in to those cravings, but we can't look back, only forward.

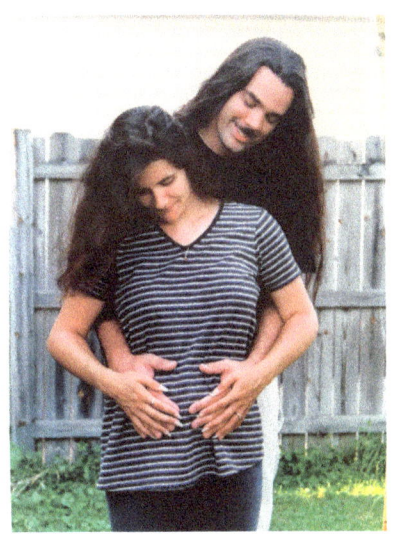

My pregnancy was not easy, but it was mine and I enjoyed every single second of it. The flutters in the beginning that became kicks later on, watching my belly and my baby move from side to side. Actually seeing a foot press against the left side of my belly and then it was definitely her bottom pressing hard as she moved about.

The sickness the whole nine months was worth all of those incredible moments I shared with her. I never had a feeling of wanting it to end, I loved every second of it and looked forward to having a natural birth. I read everything, took Lamaze classes, and even took private yoga training classes, I was beyond ready.

In one of my last appointments, when I returned home, I started bleeding. Every time I called my doctors I was told it was normal and they would see me in a few days. I continued to pray, and believe everything would be just fine. But when they saw me at my next appointment I could tell immediately not everything was normal. They told me there were a lot of signs of stress with my baby, and this type of bleeding was not the normal they had thought.

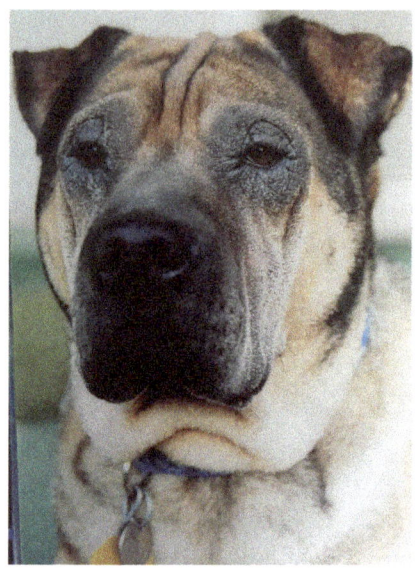

So we were told to head right to the hospital, as I said before this was July and our first baby was at home, our dog, Shar.

    We did not have air-conditioning and it was going to be in the nineties that beautiful Wednesday, and Shar needed to go to Grandma and Grandpa's house. We stopped home, which was on the way to the hospital, to get her and I had a bite of the ricotta cookie I had bought at the Italian festival. I guess I wasn't supposed to eat that day but being a pregnant momma and not knowing how this day was going to go I needed a bite of something and a cookie sounded perfect. My parents met us in the parking lot of the hospital to take Shar to their house as we were admitted to the hospital. The nurses didn't believe I was pregnant let alone having a baby that day, I was tiny in their eyes.

    It didn't take long before they decided we weren't going to try to induce labor, we were being rushed in for a cesarean section, the umbilical cord had wrapped around my baby's neck but we delivered mostly fine.

    We were fighters and I gave birth to a beautiful 5 pounds and 1 ounce, 18 ¼ inch long baby girl!

LIVE NATURALLY

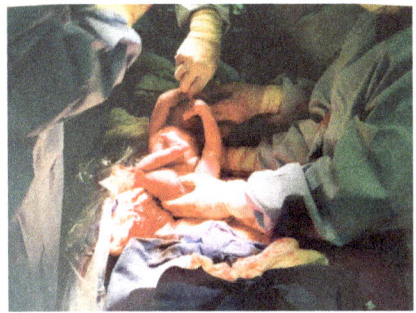 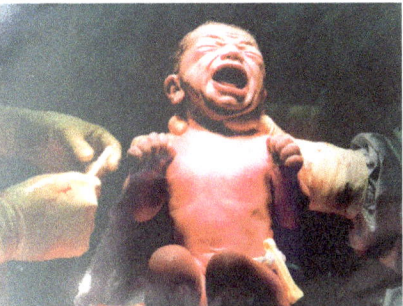

Childbirth is one of God's most amazing miracles, but there were some crazy moments, I felt hot and they pumped something in me, I felt them tugging and they pumped more in me. I kept feeling like I was going to pass out but literally refused to especially when at that point they made her father leave, I was by myself and the vibe in the room didn't feel good. The doctors stopped talking to me and just did their job so I started talking to myself and my Lord that everything was fine and this had to be over soon.

Thankfully, it was, they wheeled me past the nursery to show me my daughter through the window and then into my room where they realized someone didn't take the bed out of the room and now I would have to get myself from the bed I was in to the bed in the room. Really? So, I am numb from the waist down and have just had major surgery, they told me I had to go slow and I told them I don't do anything slow and that's not happening. The nurses said they never saw a woman pull herself that fast and then they pumped me with more medication and I passed out.

When I woke and saw my family, I asked where our baby was and they said in the nursery still, I told them to please go get her and make them stop pumping me with medication, I could not take that and would rather deal with the pain.

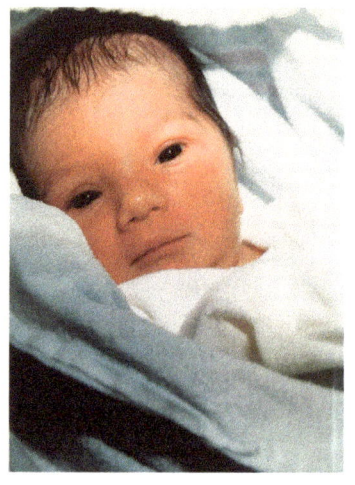

Seeing her tiny little body staring up at me was amazing, being the photographer that I am, I laid her on my legs and took her picture, the nurses said they never saw a baby that little and so aware of her surroundings. Yes, she was born a few weeks early but I think she was ready to see the world!

Our first meeting. I will never forget those beautiful brown eyes looking up at me. This tiny little girl that her father and I created. "Hi, baby girl, I'm your momma and nothing will ever take me away from you!"

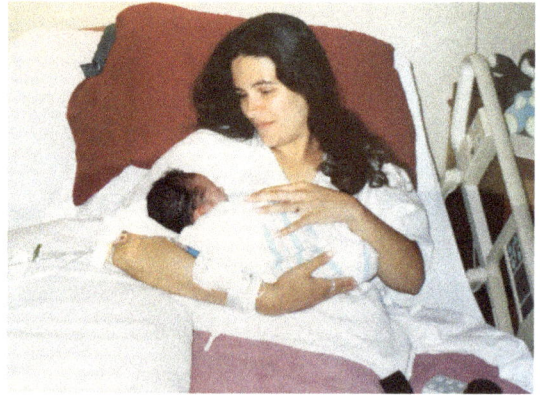

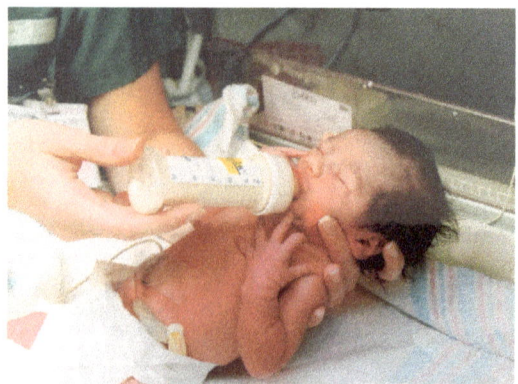

With everything I was going through and the medications they had been pumping into me against my wishes, they said I could not breastfeed and they had already tried giving her formula while I was still in surgery.

She refused it that first day but in the end that was what her first food was, *ugh,* not what I had wanted and especially because it didn't agree with her little tummy, it became soy formula. At the time soy was this amazing all-natural food, you did not hear of or know about Monsanto or GMOs. I know I said this before but boy, do I ever wish I knew then what I know now because I don't like the idea that I made sure all the foods I introduced my daughter to were all natural and organic except for her first food in this world.

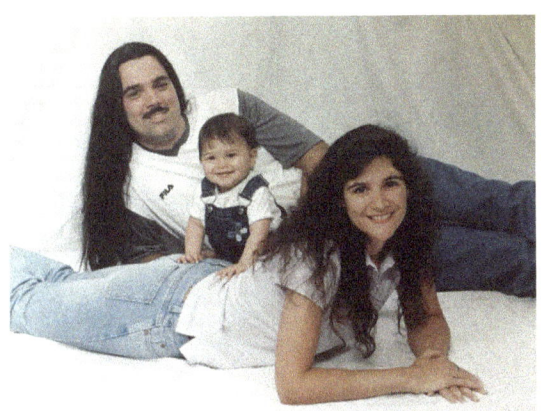

I am proud to say that my daughter has never eaten fast food, not a hamburger, not a hot dog, not even taco meat. Actually, not any form of red meat at all.

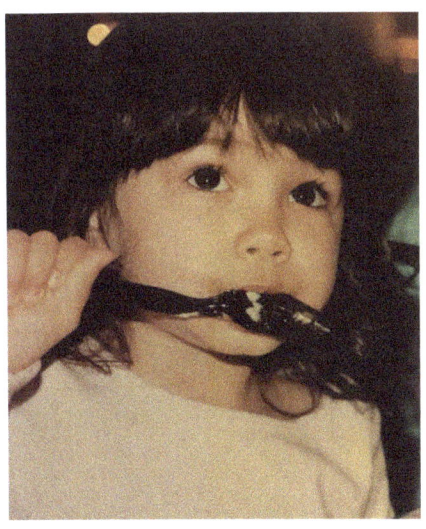

My dad's favorite story to tell is how he had taken her downtown to watch the boats and asked her at three years old if she wanted to get a hot dog with him at the little restaurant there, and she told him how bad hot dogs were for you and you should not eat them.

He said, "I couldn't believe it, you sure did teach her well, because that day I didn't get a hot dog and yes, they are not good for you but for some reason taste good." Ha ha. My dad, he thinks of food much better now than he used to!

My daughter and I do, on occasion, eat chicken, turkey, and salmon but all our meats are wild, unprocessed, and aren't fed any antibiotics. I make sure all of the fruits and vegetables I purchase are organic and mostly from local farmers. I try very hard to limit our breads and flours but if I do purchase bread I make sure no gluten is added and it has five ingredients or less. Ever since the fat-free phase of our lives, I don't buy into labeling, I read ingredient lists. To me it's easy, if I can't pronounce it, I won't eat it, and neither will my family. If it has a huge ingredient list to make its shelf life stable, I won't buy it. This goes for everything I buy not only food but for every product in my house I go by the same principle.

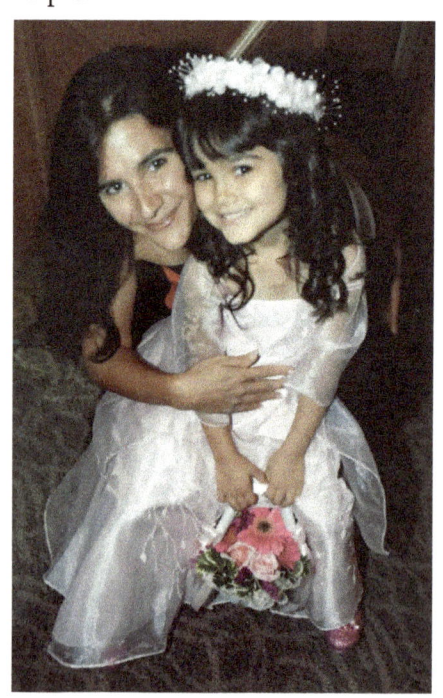

It's not easy raising a child that sees her friends eating things that I won't buy. So at a young age, if she saw something in the store, instead of saying "no," I would read the ingredient list and explain the good ingredients and the bad ingredients. Then we would figure out a way to make it ourselves.

I have caught a lot of flack the past twenty plus years, about what I would buy, what I would eat, and what I would feed my family. I had family members and friends literally mad at me for the way I was raising my family, and some turned away from us. It is funny to me that now so many have jumped on board and have opened their eyes to what has happened to our food, skincare, and medical industries.

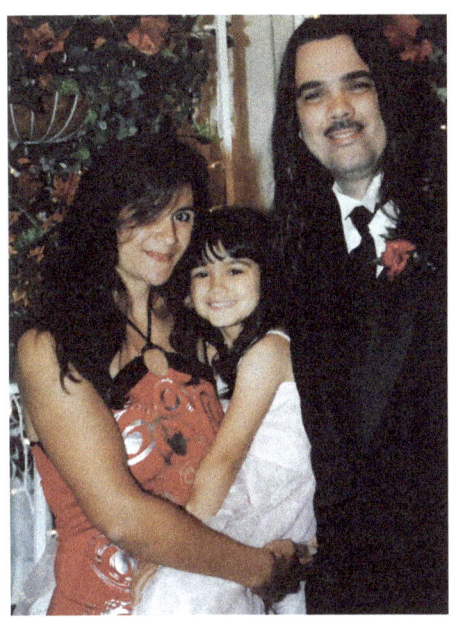

I will never say I am perfect. I am forever learning and experimenting. When raising a child, sometimes you do what others have told you to do, for example, vaccines and medications. But as we have raised our daughter, I would try homeopathic remedies first before medications, some may take longer to work, and some may work right away. Some we adapted into our lifestyle to stay healthy so we won't get sick.

At the time of my cancer diagnosis, the doctors couldn't explain how my cells changed, they burned a part of my cervix, which at that time I didn't understand but let them do. I know my prayers were answered, I know my daughter and I were saved by our Lord for a reason bigger than we know. I know we were meant to be here longer than the doctors at that time thought we would be. So ever since the cancer diagnosis, I really have paid attention to our food and skincare products, I am diligent about what we use in our household and stay away from a lot of products on purpose. Over the years, I have created our own products to try to stay as healthy as we possibly can be. And we continue to be a family built on faith and trust in our Lord.

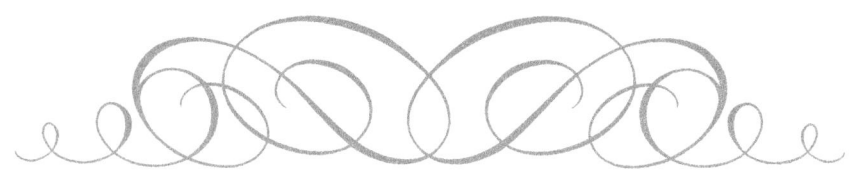

Where We Were

I will *walk by faith* even when I cannot *see*.

—2 Corinthians 5:7

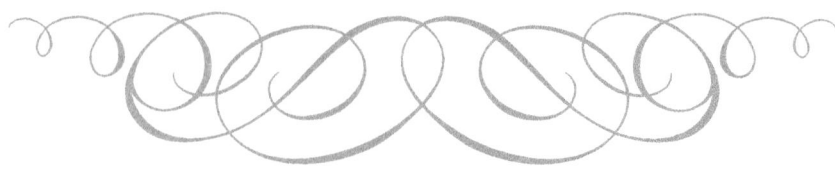

LIVE NATURALLY

This is something not easy for me to write about, let alone talk about. I have a story I don't know how to tell, and so let me say it this way.

Hi! How are you?

Four simple words we say often to each other every day but do we ever answer it truthfully?

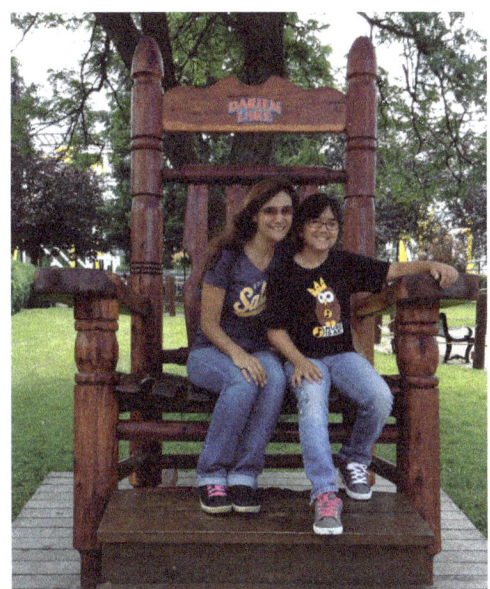

For the most part I am good. The most important thing to me is my faith and my family. God has always had me in the palm of his hands even when I couldn't see the light through my darkest hours. And my family stood by me and continues to through this journey.

So, yes, when I answer, "I am good, how are you?"

This is me being truthful.

Have you ever hit your head?

Have you ever hit your head so hard that you felt your neck snap inside your body? Not snap like crack, but almost feel like it bent backward and downward into your body.

Well, unfortunately, I did, it was June of 2013, I was working my second night job and the show was over, I was ready to go home. I quickly started grabbing all the glassware I could and after many trips did the same routine but this one I hit the top of my head against the two by four end of the bar, I totally misjudged my steps. I hit it like a bull drives his head through the red cape, except this wasn't a cape, this was wood. I should have passed out right there but instead willed myself not to because of the glassware that I was still holding.

I could not think and felt like I was going to throw up, nauseous, dizzy, and falling into a tunnel vision. I willed myself not to black out, surprisingly it worked—there is something to say about mind over matter for sure. I rushed into the bathroom where I started to black out and now I was alone. I rushed back out and grabbed ice for my head and told anyone that would listen what happened. My words started to sound garbled and my sight very foggy and slow, it didn't feel real and no one was concerned. Your shift is not done, there is work to still do . . . somehow I fought through it, I have no idea how, I don't remember much after that and now it is too late. I feel crazy telling my man what happened to me. I have a drink to relax but now it sounds like I have had more than one even though I haven't. It's a concussion, the hospital won't help and it's late, I can't sit in a hospital and I have to work the next day, time to sleep but should I? You shouldn't with a concussion but I have to, I have to be at my real job in a few hours and I am a mom, I need to be okay to get my daughter off to school in a few hours. The pain is excruciating, and I can't think straight.

How crazy that I can remember half of that night maybe because of trying to tell so many that night what was going on, and writing it down to remember to tell the doctors in the months after as well. But the months that followed I don't remember much except through pictures.

The pains of a concussion don't happen all at once, it happens over time and can't always be seen or understood by others. Depending on who surrounds you, you may have people argue with you and walk away from you. This makes your journey so much harder and lonelier.

But you will find your true family and friends that love you and stand by you through it all.

I had all of these.

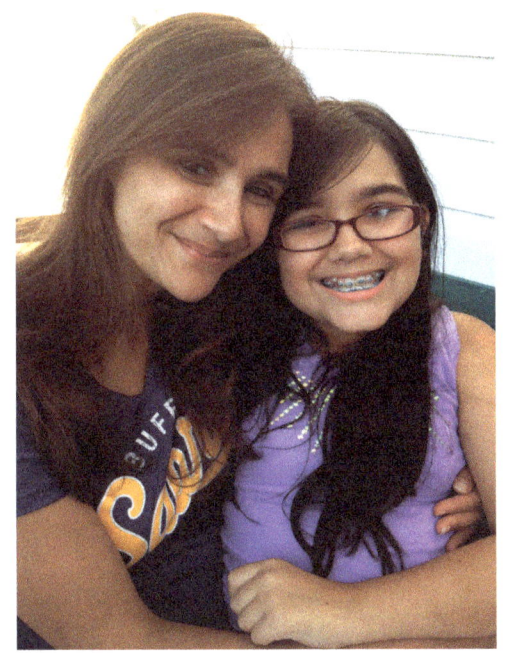

    I blamed myself a lot. First off, it was my carelessness that caused me to hit my head. I also felt maybe it happened to me for a reason, I was working all the time—two jobs most times, sixty plus hours a week—most of my time is at work, not at home with my family, maybe I was being told to slow down, that wasn't my path. My path in this life is greater than working that hard all the time for someone else's path all for extra money. Life is not about money.

    In the weeks and months that followed I lost feeling on my left side. I was in constant pain from the top of my head to the bottom of my feet. I called myself a train wreck of a spine, but in reality it was true. My neck healed to the right and my lower back healed to the left and twisted my nerves up in tangles. I could not sit and I could not sleep, when I did I had to be propped up and pillows under my knees and I would still wake numb everywhere. I was told when I did sleep I would stop breathing and then gasp for air. It was extremely scary and then my memory started to slip and I would slur my words and drop things.

The memory loss and walking in a cloudlike state were my first ills that lasted so long and still linger. Then three months after, my body gave up, I could not move or bend. My left side of my body would go numb. Excruciating pain does not even begin to explain. I cannot explain it because it is all so internal, people look at you and you walk and talk and make excuses if you slur your words so no one understands not even doctors. You can only cover for yourself and argue your way out of things so much before you finally crack and need help.

Doctors didn't help at that time, they told me concussions could take anywhere from two months to two years to heal, which is correct, but sometimes depending on where you hit your head, things can get really bad before they ever get better. Unfortunately, that was me six months after my concussion. I was told by my doctor she thought I had Multiple Sclerosis (MS) so finally would send me for an MRI. She was wrong, and the neurologist only offered me pain meds and psychiatric meds since they didn't find any lesions for Multiple Sclerosis (MS). The way the medical industry works is they offer you medication for the pain and since they cannot figure out what you are going through, they want to give you medication in case you start to get depressed.

I refused this. I am a natural mom and would rather feel the pain than mask it and find a natural way to heal my body. By telling them this, they wrote in my records that I refused treatment and that I was moving. Funny how when you want to truly find a cure for your ailments and pain you are deemed unreasonable and therefore unwanted.

When things seem bleak they tend to get worse before they get better, the injury site seemed to be a magnet for some reason. I got hit in that exact spot on two different occasions while at my daughter's volleyball games. I could not attend the practices any longer because it seemed every time I was there, a ball would come barreling at my head. And yes, I even took a basketball to the head while hosting my daughter's birthday party.

When you reinjure yourself it is like it has happened all over again—the excruciating pain, nausea, dizziness, and inability to see straight is something you cannot understand unless you have gone through it.

My doctors at the time didn't believe most of my ailments because I hit the top of my head, they told me the injuries I was experiencing should only happen to someone if they hit the sides of their head. At one point I had a PA push me down on the table by my chest because I wasn't laying down fast enough right after I had explained to her that my neck was out and I had just gone to the chiropractor the day before. After that I could not sit up and wound up back at my chiropractor. A lot of my eye sight problems that happened after the concussion I was told comes with age and was normal, it seemed like there was always a reason that came back to me making up what I was going through.

Until I finally got a second opinion from a new neurologist, he is a neurologist that sees a lot of MS patients and now only sees MS patients. But when he saw me and looked closer at my injuries, he informed me that they are realizing more with the brain, and technically I have a brain injury that resembles with a football player, the difference with me and a football player is they wear helmets and I didn't.

I may always have some issues from it but I have come a long way from where I once was.

Concussions and brain injuries are injuries that the people around you cannot understand no matter how hard they try. You don't have any physical outward injuries that people can see, everything is internal—you walk, well, kind of, and you talk, you may slur a bit but in some cases, like me, you try to cover that up. You start to forget everything, for me, I am a photographer and I thank the Lord for that because if someone asked me something I truly didn't remember, I would go back through my photos to remind myself.

So, now what? Where do you turn when you are trying to heal yourself naturally?

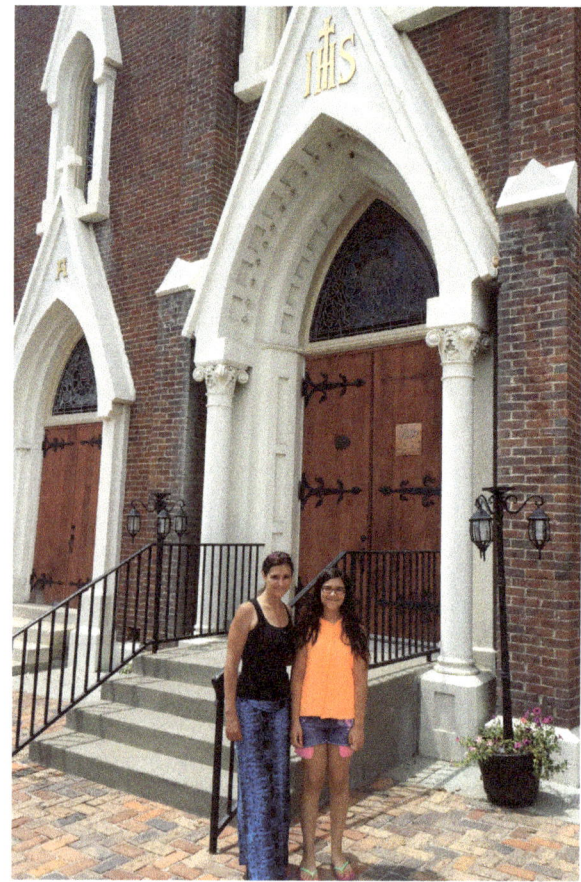

Well, for me, it's a lot of things—my faith, my family, exercise, and nutrition. But it became much more than I ever thought it would. Things I didn't exactly know about before this injury.

I have a friend who is a chiropractor so after many talks he talked me into chiropractic care. He was my saving grace so I didn't lose my main job, and I got function back in my body. I could feel and use my left side, I wasn't in constant pain anymore, but after two and a half years of care from him I still had many ailments.

What are they, you ask?

I still had memory issues, walking in a cloudlike state, thyroid type issues, insomnia more often than I would care to admit, nightmares if I slept, I never want those ever again and panic I never wanted to admit nor talk about. My vision, they say, is normal but the way I see and the processing of what I see is not normal.

Traumas can come in many forms, not only hits to the head, you don't realize how much you hold on to until it all comes to a head.

My next step is Brain Core Therapy, what is that, you may ask. Well, to me this is the most amazing noninvasive treatment that anyone with brain trauma, learning disabilities, memory loss, migraines, anxiety, depression, insomnia, ADHD, PTSD, autism, or just to keep your brain at its peak performance, can have.

You exercise your body why not your brain?

When I truly started listening to my friend and his wife, I realized I had been going through four to six reasons why to try BrainCore Therapy.

Like I said, BrainCore neurofeedback is noninvasive, I won't go into major detail but it is a natural drug-free approach to reteach the brain to function in a more balanced healthy way. I was skeptical for some crazy reason, probably more so because I couldn't think straight for the near year we had all spoken about it.

But with my healthy lifestyle, I knew this brain injury was heading me closer to a life similar to Alzheimer's and I wasn't willing at my young age to keep losing myself, I needed to get myself back.

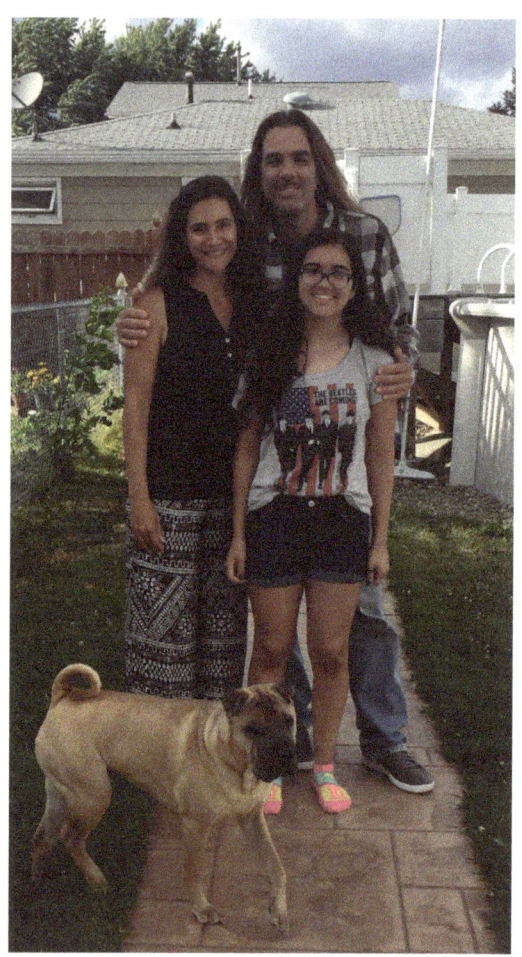

And I have, I know, I still have extra treatments to do, and now feel why in the heck isn't everyone doing this? We live in a very fast-paced society and we need help to retrain our brain just like we tune up our cars. I work in special education and have an extremely strong feeling this could and would help some if not all of my students, but I cannot push my thoughts on parents nor do I really know the parents so I need to be silent as to this amazing treatment that could help so many.

Neurofeedback is not new, it has been around for probably forty years but it has come a long way, it is as easy as you watching a movie or a TV show you enjoy and your brain finding the right way to think and unclutter itself, in the simplest way I can explain.

So how has it helped me?

Well, to begin with, ever since my concussion, I have been unable to read a book without rereading the same page five times before giving up, I lost the ability to do simple math, which is a big blow to the ego of an accounting major. And I would have never, in a million years, been able to write out my thoughts, let alone organize them and create this book.

Besides all of these reasons, the insomnia is something of the past, and thankfully the nightmares stopped. The migraines I didn't realize I was having are gone, the depression of not being able to think is gone and I will never feel that again. I was at a point I didn't know how it felt to not be an anxious person, how fast we forget who we are.

I am happy to say I am calm and feeling normal again. The memory loss, most has come back, some hasn't, but that is okay, almost daily something new pops in and others around me notice the improvements.

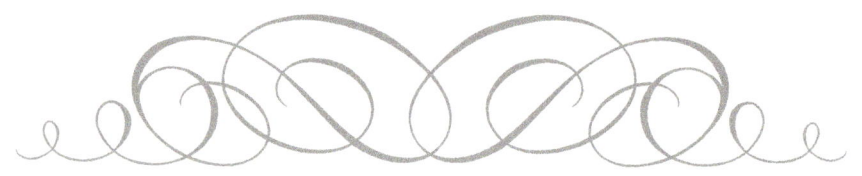

My Theories

The phrase *"Do not be Afraid"* is written in the bible 365 times. That's a daily reminder from God to live every day being fearless.

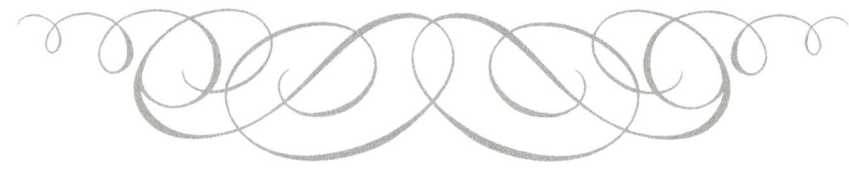

I call all of what I do my theories. I have read a ton throughout my lifetime and have tried many different ways of living a healthy lifestyle. Some things I have tried if they didn't work I won't continue but there are theories that have worked for me and I continue to do them today. I never push these theories on others, we are all unique and some things that work for me may not work for you and some things that work for you may not work for me. That is why I call them theories, because nothing is set in stone that this is what you need to do to stay healthy. If you are interested in testing your body and seeing what it takes to have your body live a healthy lifestyle, I encourage you to try some of the things I have, but if you are not interested that is okay with me. That is what makes us all individuals and unique!

In the pages that follow you will see what I feed my family and how easy it can be to live an organic all-natural lifestyle. Most of my meals do not have a lot of ingredients, I try to make things as easy as possible. You will see nothing is crazy exotic, it may actually be something you make at home but a different version of it. Like I said, when raising a family we also would like something that may not be the healthiest for our bodies so my job has become figuring out how to make a better version of it.

You will notice in my recipes I use organic unsweetened almond milk instead of milk, this is an easy alternative, the measurements will always be the same. And the taste will never vary, if you are new to almond milk this will be an easy way for you to learn how to use it and to see that you can easily swap it for cow's milk.

The other thing you will notice is instead of flour, I may use garbanzo bean flour. This is another easy swap, the measurements will stay the same and the taste will never vary from a recipe that calls for flour. You will notice a few recipes I still call for flour, which is because it is a recipe I do not make often and haven't gotten to try it yet, but I know it will taste exactly the same. But for the reason that I have not done it myself, I will not push it on others and if you are unsure you can use regular flour.

I do not have a sweet tooth, so when I make something that needs sugar I always cut back on the measurements. The recipes I have written that call for sugar are the true measurements, if you are like me and don't like using a lot of sugar, follow the recipe the first time and decide if you would like to cut back, go for it! I have cut back a bit and my recipes tend to taste the same and no one can tell the difference.

I do use cheeses and will never claim to be completely vegan. But the thing I always do when purchasing cheese is inform myself how it is made, processed, and treated. I buy most of my cheeses from organic farmers that will never use antibiotics on their animals and allow their animals free range of their pastures.

I rarely eat animals but when I do I make sure I know how they are treated, an easy thing I think about is what that animal ate, I will have eaten too. I do not want to eat an animal that has been pumped with antibiotics and fed food that in nature it would not normally eat. An animal should live a life and not be confined to a pen with so many others, if I had my complete choice, I would not eat animal products at all, this is something I go back and forth on all the time. I will go months without eating any form of an animal and then I will eat fish or chicken on occasion. Sometimes my body needs that protein and sometimes it doesn't. This is a personal choice for everyone individually, and I do not pass judgment on anyone and hope no one will pass judgment on me.

Ever since my pregnancy I have not been able to tolerate eggs, so when I cook I have a way to substitute eggs with flax seed.

It works well with pancakes, quick breads, brownies, muffins, cookies, and many other recipes.

Flax Egg

1 tbsp. flaxseed meal
2 1/2 tbsps. water

Let rest for 5 minutes to thicken and use in replacement of 1 egg.

I won't include it in every recipe I share with you but know that all of my ingredients are organic or from an organic farm. I tend to cook meals by the season, if they are fresh and readily available, I use them in some amazing recipes. If something is out of season but I can get it frozen and still be organic, I will make these recipes too. I suggest when following my recipes, you chose the same high quality ingredients. When you shop for produce look at the numbers, there is a way to know if a produce is conventional, organic, or genetically engineered (GMO).

- If it is five digits beginning with a nine, it is organic, this is what I purchase.
- If it is four digits beginning with a four, it is conventional, nonorganic, and pesticides are used.
- If it is five digits and beginning with an eight, it is genetically modified (GMO).

I know in our society this can be a bit pricey but you can watch prices and shop at farmer's markets also. I invest in a local organic farm in my area, this is a great way to help the farmers in your area and the environment by buying local and reducing your carbon footprint.

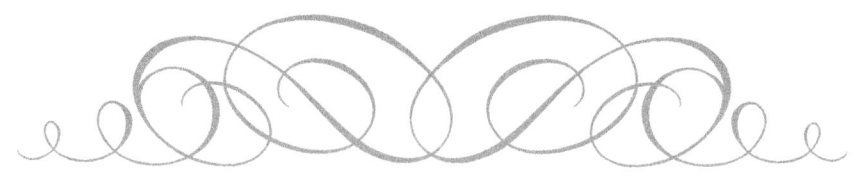

My Recipes

She is clothed in *Strength* and *Dignity*,
and she *Laughs* without fear of the future.

—Proverbs 31:25

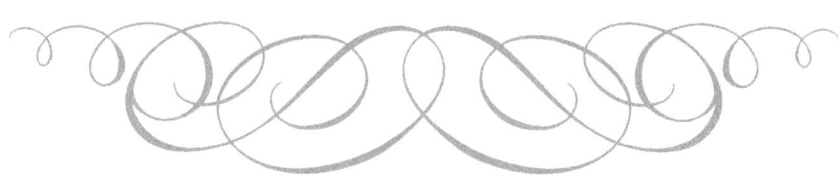

In the next pages you are going to find out how much I love to cook and feed my family and friends. Everyone tells me it's easy for me because I love to cook, and I know a lot of people that don't love to cook, so cooking seems extremely hard for them.

No one ever taught me how to cook. I started at nine years old helping the family. I would have things prepped for me to basically heat through one night or so a week. Then at probably twelve or thirteen, when I had my paper route, my dad and I would cook everyone breakfast since we would be up so early on Sunday mornings. Actually, after we would be done delivering papers my dad would take me out to breakfast, but when the family found out we were going out to breakfast they weren't too happy. Ha ha. Our answer was, "Then get up and deliver papers with us," which no one was interested in, so we started going shopping and preparing breakfasts for them as they would rise from the smell of our food!

This is how I started, but in later years when I was on my own, I really needed to teach myself especially because of how my tastes and thoughts on food were ever changing. But being on your own and running your own household, sometimes more intense exotic recipes are not in the budget. So, my cooking became somewhat simple in my mind anyways. Nothing is too difficult and nothing calls for crazy ingredients.

My hope in you reading and trying my recipes is that you will find cooking easier and find a love that I have.

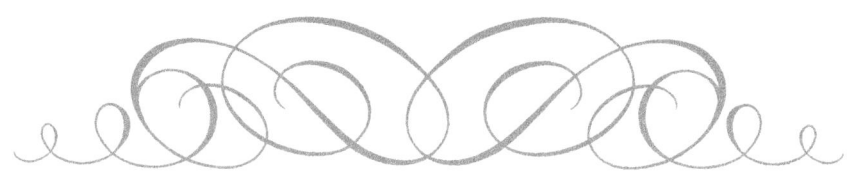

Breakfast

Bless the *Food* before us,
The *Family* beside us,
and the *Love* between us.
                Amen.

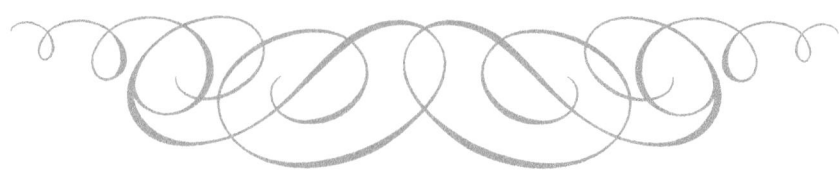

What do you think of when you think of breakfast foods? Most people think bagels, pancakes, waffles, oatmeal, eggs, home fries, fruit, sausage, bacon, or how about breakfast pizza.

Let's look at that list . . . carbs and sugars mostly, not a great way to start your day. In reality, this type of a breakfast may actually make you crash and crave other unhealthy foods throughout your morning. But isn't breakfast the most important meal of the day? *Hmmm,* actually no, Mr. Kellogg said that saying when he started making cornflakes cereal. If you like looking up history or documentaries, look up Mr. Kellogg, you will never look at breakfast cereal the same again.

In reality, the farmers for centuries have it right, they would wake up, work in the fields, and work up an appetite. So lunch would actually be the most important meal of their days. My dad even tells me my ancestors did the same, but it was the women—his aunts would wake up and tend to their gardens and the first thing they would have every morning was their coffee with a bit of liquor added for a quick pick-me-up. Ha ha. Too funny!

Now you may be thinking that my family must not eat breakfast. No, this is not true, we are Americans and have been raised with different habits, but have adopted our own. Each of us is a little different. My daughter always has a piece of fruit before she heads out to school. She does not like my protein shakes so this works for her, sometimes she will have a kefir smoothie before heading out the door instead. For us it is a protein shake. Myself I tend to have my ACV water after I wake and usually wait 3 hours or so before having my shake for breakfast.

But on different occasions I do make big breakfasts for my family, Easter and Christmas are my main days to really dive into my breakfast recipes. And for every holiday I make a different fruit tray, here are a few of them, aren't they cute! They don't last long as this is what I serve my family and friends while I am cooking the rest of our meal.

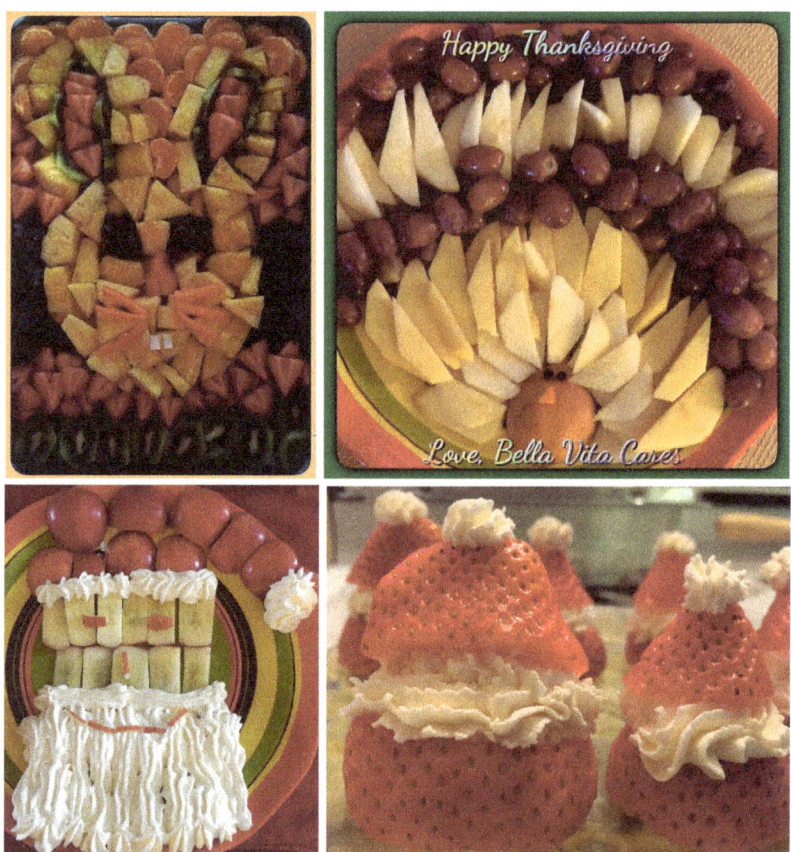

I have very strong opinions as to the order of how our bodies should eat. For example, fruits break down the quickest of all foods and is out of the stomach in twenty to thirty minutes. It is extremely important to eat an alkaline food, either ripe fruit or raw vegetable at each meal first, on an empty stomach.

I know, now your saying, "What, now I have to retrain my family and myself on an order of how we eat?"

No, I will never push my theories on anyone but if you wanted to try some, this is an easy one and you can start with my holiday fruit trays. I have these beautifully displayed after we come home from church so my family unknowingly is doing something extremely healthy for their bodies. And by starting your meal like this, it gives the perfect rest time in between and helps prevent you from overeating.

So, if I have interested you with this theory, then I am sure you're now wondering how to do this with your daily meals. Again, simple adjustments—serve a salad prior to your meal or offer raw veggies while you are preparing lunch or dinner. This seriously became an easy adjustment for my family, there wasn't any forcing but everyone eats all their veggies prior to any protein on their plates. I never forced anyone in my family to do this, it just became natural. If you don't think too much about it and just try it, it can become natural for you too!

So here are some of my family's favorites I serve for breakfast.

Kefir Smoothie

1 cup blueberries, frozen
2 cups kefir, plain organic
1 tsp. raw honey

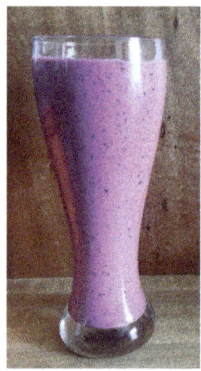

Blend all ingredients together.
This will serve one for breakfast or two for a prebreakfast served with eggs and vegetables.
Any berry works for this recipe. I use frozen because they are available all year and then I do not need to add ice.
My go-to smoothie to keep everyone healthy!

Andrea's Easy on the Go

1 scoop chocolate protein powder
2 tsps. ground flaxseed
4–5 ice cubes
25 oz. water

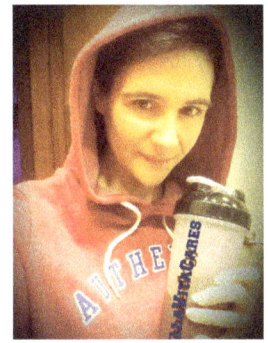

Shake and go!
To use what I use go to my website: www.bellavitacares.com.

Cinnamon Roll

1 serving chocolate protein powder
1 cup nonfat milk or almond milk
1 tsp. ground cinnamon
1 tsp. vanilla extract

For the best taste experience, use a blender and add ice. The more ice, the thicker it gets. The more milk, the creamier it gets!
To use what I use go to my website: www.bellavitacares.com.

Healthy Fat Shake

(That Keeps You Full Longer)

1 scoop chocolate protein powder
1 tbsp. ground flaxseeds
1 tsp. coconut oil
1 tsp. almond butter
1 tsp. ground turmeric
1 tsp cinnamon, nutmeg
and chai seasoning mix
2 cups water

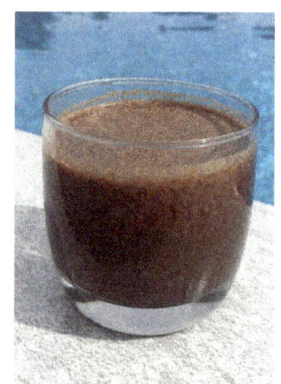

Blend and once blended transfer the mixture to a larger shaker cup and rinse the blender cup with 1 more cup of water, now add that water to the larger shaker cup. Put the lid on and shake well. Your drink will be about 25 ounces, enjoy!

To use what I use go to my website: www.bellavitacares.com.

Monkey Heaven

1 scoop chocolate protein powder
1/2 cup unsweetened almond milk
1/2 cup frozen banana
1/2 cup water
1 tbsp. peanut butter
1 1/2 cup ice

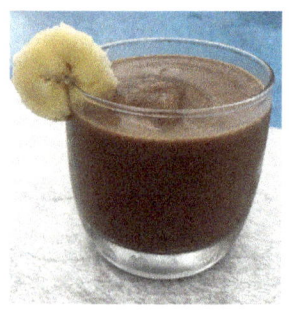

Blend and enjoy!
To use what I use go to my website: www.bellavitacares.com.

Thin Mintalicious

1 scoop chocolate protein powder
1 tsp. mint extract
1 cup unsweetened almond milk
ice
Blend and enjoy!
To use what I use go to my website: www.bellavitacares.com.

Berry-Licious

1 cup unsweetened almond milk
1 scoop strawberry protein powder
1 cup fresh or frozen raspberries
1 cup ice

Blend until smooth.
To use what I use go to my website: www.bellavitacares.com.

Nuts About Berries

1 cup unsweetened almond milk
1 scoop strawberry protein powder
1/2 cup fresh or frozen blackberries
2 tbsps. chopped raw pecans
1 cup ice

Blend until smooth.
To use what I use go to my website: www.bellavitacares.com.

Banana Milkshake

1 scoop vanilla protein powder
1 banana (or 1 1/2 for more banana flavor)
1/2 cup ice
1/2 cup water

Blend and enjoy!

Banana Nut Shake

1 scoop vanilla protein powder
1/2 cup unsweetened almond milk
1/2 cup frozen banana
1/2 cup water
1 tbsp. peanut butter
1 1/2 cup ice

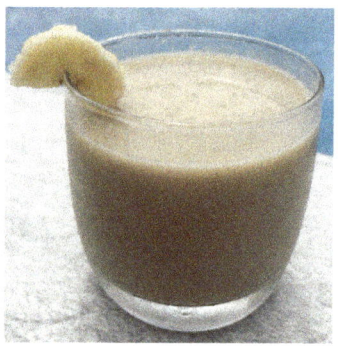

Blend and enjoy!
To use what I use go to my website: www.bellavitacares.com.

Café Latte

1 scoop vanilla protein powder
1/2 cup unsweetened almond milk
1/2 cup brewed coffee, cooled
1 tsp. unsweetened cocoa, 100% cocoa
1/2 cup ice

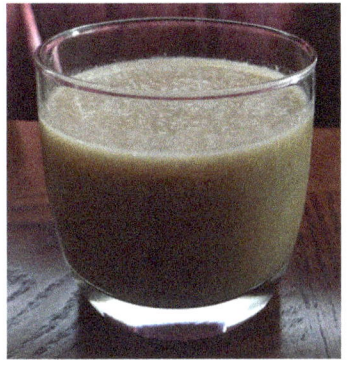

Blend and enjoy!
To use what I use go to my website: www.bellavitacares.com.

Iced Mocha

1 scoop vanilla protein powder
1 tsp. flaxseeds, ground
1 tsp. coconut oil
1/2 cup brewed coffee, cooled
1 cup filtered water

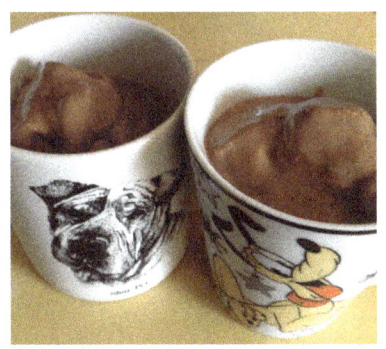

Blend until smooth.
To use what I use go to my website: www.bellavitacares.com.

Neapolitan

1 cup water
1 scoop vanilla protein powder
1/2 cup strawberries, frozen
1 tsp. unsweetened cocoa powder
1 cup ice

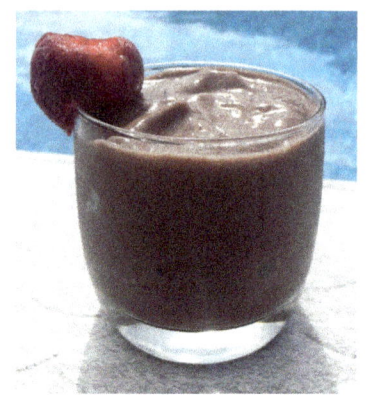

Blend until smooth.
Add 1/2 of a banana to make it a banana split!
To use what I use go to my website: www.bellavitacares.com.

Vanilla Chai

1 serving vanilla protein powder
1 cup brewed chai tea
1 tsp. raw honey
1–2 cups ice

Blend until smooth.

To use what I use go to my website: www.bellavitacares.com.

Avocado Toast

1 avocado, cut in slices
4–6 slices organic rosemary bakery bread

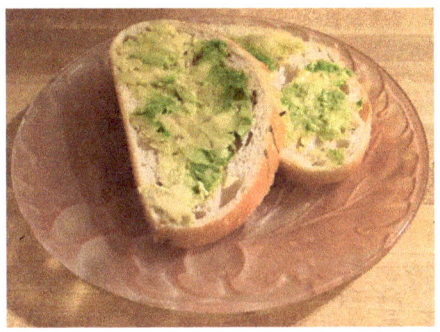

Cut and slice avocado while you are toasting your bread. Once toasted, put a few slices of avocado on each slice of bread and spread.

Something so easy can be made nutritious. As you will see from my recipes, I cannot eat a lot of these recipes as I am allergic to eggs. But I do enjoy my meals with my family, so for our holiday breakfasts, I make this along with roasted vegetables and a salad. And even though it is a breakfast, my family will eat my salads and vegetables with me! And this has become a favorite instead of toast and butter!

Broccoli Cheese Eggs or Egg Muffins

6 organic large eggs
1/4 cup almond milk
1/2 cup frozen broccoli, chopped
1/4 cup sharp cheddar cheese, shredded
1/2 tsp. coconut oil

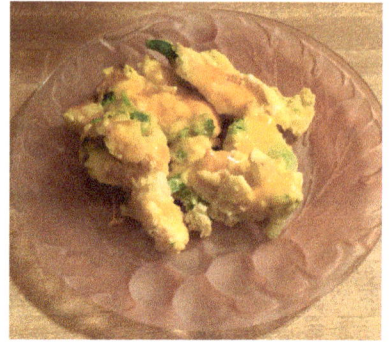

Cook in medium high heat, let coconut oil melt and make sure it covers the pan. Add egg and broccoli mixture and scramble, add shredded cheddar last after you turn off the heat and cover to allow it to melt.

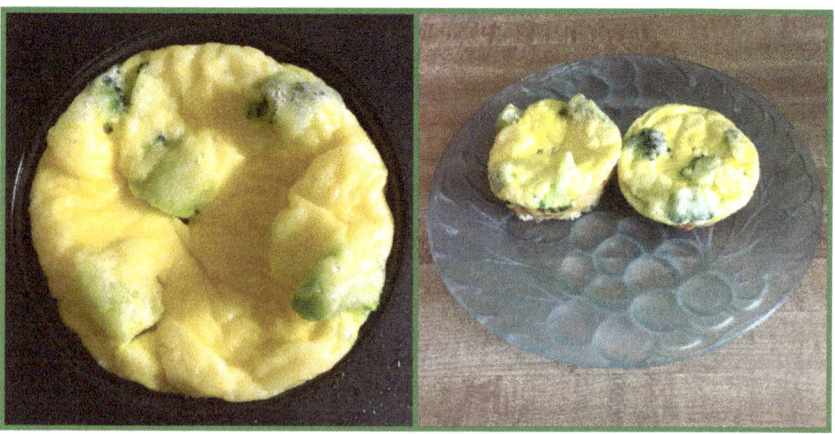

I make these egg muffins for an easy breakfast for my daughter during the week. Use coconut oil or butter to grease a muffin pan and fill them with the same mixture above, or instead of broccoli use spinach or kale. You will bake them at 350 degrees for 10–15 minutes or until cooked through. This recipe will make 6 muffins.

Cheesy Hash Brown Casserole

4 tbsp. butter
1/3 cup onion, diced
1 clove garlic, minced
4 tbsp. whole wheat flour
1 1/2 cups almond milk
2 cups extra sharp cheddar cheese, grated
1 lb. frozen hash browns, don't defrost
pepper to taste

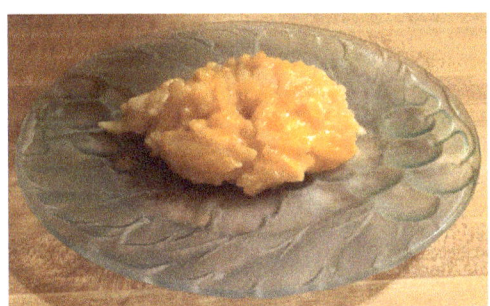

Preheat oven to 350 degrees. Grease a glass baking dish with coconut oil or olive oil. In a large sauté pan, over medium heat, melt butter. Cook the diced onion until it softens but does not brown, about 2–3 minutes. Mix in the minced garlic and cook while stirring for 1 minute.

Turn the heat down to medium low and whisk in the flour, continuously stirring until the flour darkens but does not burn, about 1–2 minutes. Whisk in the almond milk, until it is slightly thickened about 1 minute. Turn the heat off and using a spatula or wooden spoon, stir in the grated cheese until it melts. Fold in the hash browns until evenly coated.

Transfer to the baking dish being careful to push the thick mixture down on top into one even layer. Bake for 30–35 minutes uncovered, and then turn the heat up to broil for 3–4 minutes or until the top turns golden brown. Keep a close eye under the broiler so it doesn't burn. Serve warm.

This version comes out greasy. I blot the top before serving.

Healthier Hash Brown Bake

2 pkgs. frozen hash browns
2 onions, sliced and diced
1 1/2 cup almond milk
2 cups extra sharp cheddar
pepper to taste

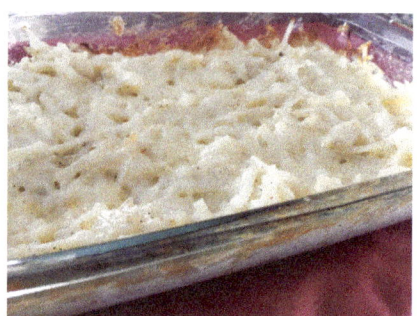

Preheat oven to 350 degrees. Grease a glass baking dish with coconut oil. Add the first package of hash browns and top with onions and 1 cup of the shredded cheese. Sprinkle 1 tsp. of black pepper on this layer before adding the second bag of hash browns.

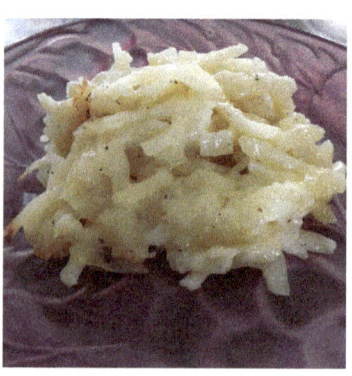

Bake for 30 minutes, you can mix it at this point but I usually don't so my onions stay in every bite. Sprinkle the last cup of cheese on the top and bake for 15 more minutes until cheese is melted.

Home Fries

6 potatoes, diced
2 red peppers, diced
2 onions, diced

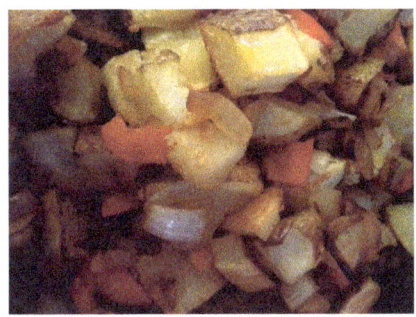

    Boil the diced potatoes on medium heat for 25 minutes. They will be still firm, drain and get them ready to fry with the diced peppers and onions.

    I use a cast iron flat top so therefore I do not use oil but if I use a frying pan, I coat my potatoes and vegetables in olive oil before frying so they don't stick.

    You will continually toss and flip them with your spatula for about 10 minutes until they are browned but not burned.

    Depending on the size of your pan, you can do these in smaller batches.

My Homemade Pancake Mix

5 cups whole wheat flour
3 cups unbleached all-purpose flour
1/2 cup sugar
2 1/2 tbsp. baking powder
4 tsps. baking soda
4 tsps. salt

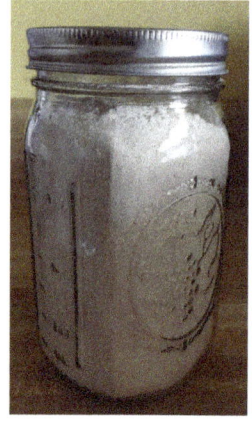

Mix together and store in an airtight container.

Blueberry Pancakes

1 cup mix
1 cup almond milk
1 egg
2 tbsp. apple sauce or olive oil

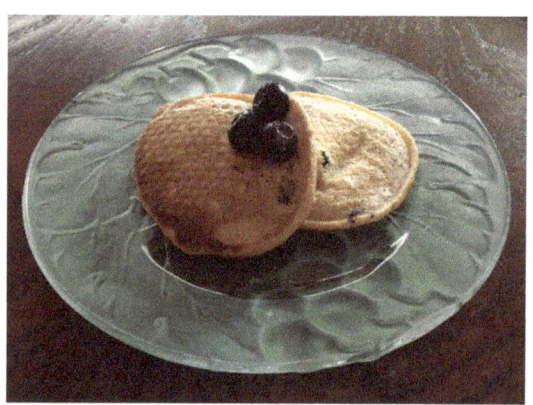

Mix together and fry in 1 tsp. coconut oil. I add 4 blueberries to each mini pancake. I make 4 at a time and this recipe makes 17.

Chocolate Chip Pancakes

1 1/2 cups pancake mix
1 1/4 cups kefir
2 eggs, lightly beaten
1 tsp. vanilla

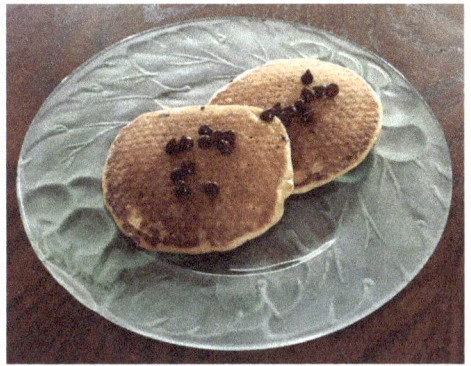

Mix together and fry in 1 tsp. coconut oil. The chocolate chips I use are soy free, nut free, dairy free, and gluten free.

Gluten-Free Buckwheat Kefir Pancakes

1 1/2 cups buckwheat flour
1 1/4 cups cultured milk kefir
 (feel free to try other kefirs)
2 eggs, lightly beaten
1/2 tsp. sea salt (optional)
1/2 tsp. baking soda
1/2 tsp. baking powder
1/2 tsp. vanilla extract
coconut oil or butter to fry

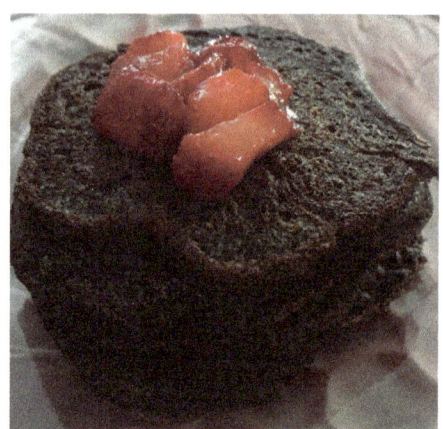

Mix flour and kefir until flour is well moistened. Cover and soak at room temperature for 24 hours.

The soaking process helps break down the grains, making the pancakes softer and the grain digestible.

In the morning, preheat the pan; mix all the other ingredients into the buckwheat mixture. At this point, it may be very bubbly, like a sourdough starter. Stir it down a bit, just to take a little air out of the batter.

Make and flip like regular pancakes.

Yogurt Parfait

1 5 oz. plain Greek yogurt
1 cup blueberries, frozen
1 tsp. flaxseed, ground

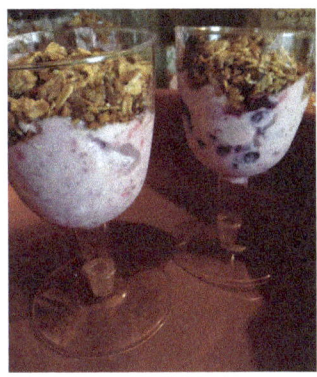

    Mix all ingredients and let sit 2–3 minutes, now with the side of a spoon, mash the blueberries. This will taste like a treat more so than a breakfast.

    You can top with my granola.

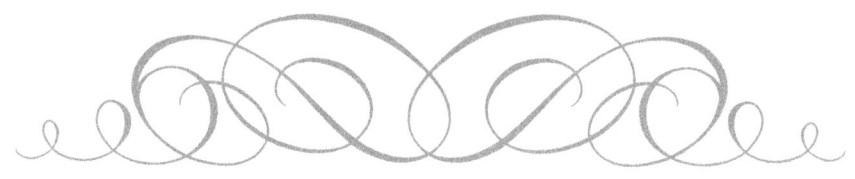

Soups

I give you thanks that I am *Fearfully, Wonderfully* made; Wonderful are your Works. My *Soul* also you knew full well.

—Psalms 139:14

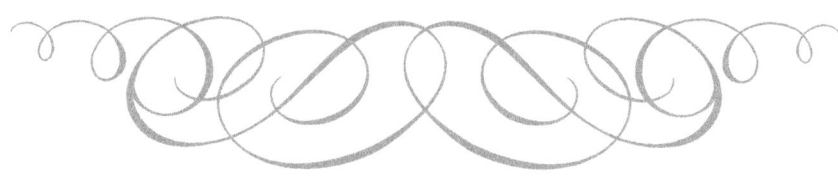

Now I am going to breakdown my most common meals in categories. You will notice my recipes tend to feed six even though we are a family of three. I try to make things easy on myself. When preparing dinners, I always make more for lunches the next day. First, I am Italian and we love to cook and feed our families so it is easy to cook more than what is needed at a meal, but this is where there is no way you can overeat—there aren't any seconds because that is always lunch the following day. And if you are like my family, if you really love a meal, you want leftovers the following day!

I don't create family style meals except on holidays, our everyday meals plate is made with the perfect amount of food and the lunches are prepared at the same time, which makes mornings run smoothly.

Also, understand that I am terrible at following directions, so if you are like me, my recipes are made with wiggle room. Don't be afraid if you didn't follow something exactly, I am sure it will come out wonderful!

What are your thoughts on soup? Is it a starter for a meal or a meal in itself? You will see from my soup recipes they easily can be a meal in itself, but sometimes I serve a basic salad prior to our soup dinners. And when I send this off to school or work the following day, it is usually paired with a fruit, raw veggies, or a salad also.

Here are my family's favorite soup recipes. I hope you enjoy them as much as we do!

Momma's Broccoli Soup

1 pkg. frozen broccoli
1 onion, chopped
4 cups vegetable broth
2 potatoes, peeled, 1" per piece
fresh ground pepper to taste
1 tbsp. olive oil

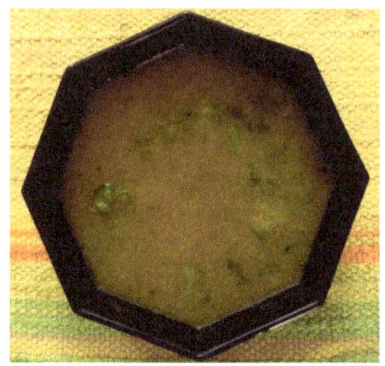

Finely chop broccoli (4 cups) and set aside. Heat oil on medium and add finely chopped onion and sweat until soft and translucent, about 10 minutes. Add stock and potatoes, bring to a boil. Reduce heat and simmer until potato is almost tender, about 12 minutes. Stir in broccoli and simmer until tender for another 10 minutes. Remove soup from heat and cool slightly before pureeing in a blender. You can leave some broccoli aside to add to the puree. Reheat a tad before serving.

I have used many different potatoes in this recipe—russet, yellow, and sweet potatoes—all work nicely.

If you are not vegan you can add grated extra sharp cheddar to garnish this soup.

Momma's Chili

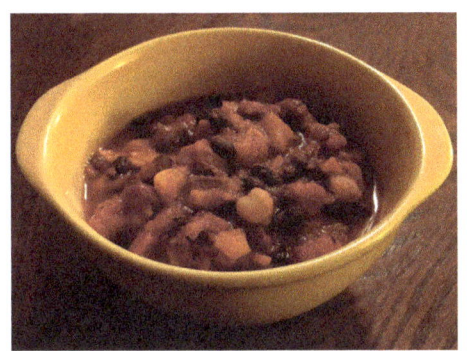

2 cans fire roasted crushed tomatoes
1 can 15 oz. black beans
1 can 15 oz. garbanzo beans
1 can 15 oz. kidney beans
1 can 15 oz. cannellini beans
1/4 red onion, diced
1 red pepper, diced
1/4–1/2 zucchini, diced
1/4–1/2 yellow squash, diced
1 large, 2 medium, 3 small garlic cloves, minced
1 1/2–2 tsp. cumin
2 tsp. Italian seasonings
1/4 tsp. cayenne, optional

Chop all of your vegetables, and drain all of your beans. Add your canned tomatoes first before your beans, and then add your veggies. Now stir.

I don't like measuring spices, it is all by the eye, and I add them to the top and make a mound in the middle.

Stir and simmer for 1–1 1/2 hours.

Taste occasionally and add spices as needed. Start with my measurements above but as it cooks you can add more, be careful though, as cayenne cooks it gets hotter. This is a very mild vegetable chili, as my daughter does not like spicy food.

Sometimes I add organic tomato paste to thicken it but it is not necessary. If you add it start with a tablespoon.

Cream of Broccoli Cauliflower Soup

3 cups broccoli
3 cups cauliflower
4 cups vegetable broth
2 tbsp. olive oil
1 clove garlic, chopped
1/4–1/2 cup onion, chopped
2 tbsp. garbanzo bean flour
2 cups almond milk
pepper to taste

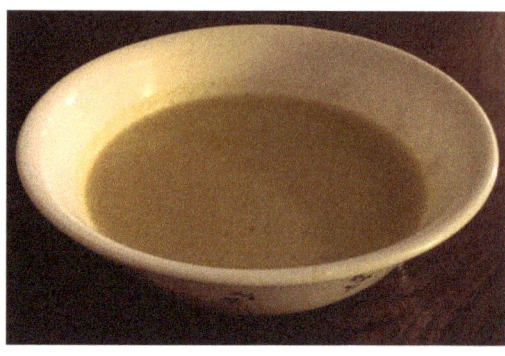

Chop broccoli and cauliflower into florets, you can use fresh or frozen if not in season. Sauté onion and garlic in 1 tsp. olive oil on medium heat for about 10 minutes or until translucent but not browned. Add broccoli and cauliflower to this mixture and pour vegetable broth over it. Cover and turn heat up to boil for 10 minutes. Once boiled and vegetables are tender when poked with a fork, take off heat to cool.

In a separate saucepan, add 2 tbsps. olive oil and garbanzo bean flour, cook on low for about 5 minutes, whisking it together. Slowly add the unsweetened almond milk and bring to a boil then simmer till thickened, stirring constantly with the whisk for 10 more minutes or so. This is important so the sauce won't get lumpy, if by chance it does it is okay because you can blend it with the soup.

Now the broccoli and cauliflower should be cooled enough to blend in your blender, start by pulsing to make sure it is cool enough. Stir the puree into the almond milk sauce and add pepper to taste. If you would like you can add sharp cheddar when serving.

Creamy Butternut Squash Soup with Quinoa

1 tbsp. butter
1 onion, chopped
4 cups vegetable broth
1 butternut squash
2 cups water
1 cup quinoa
1 tsp. cumin
1 1" piece of ginger

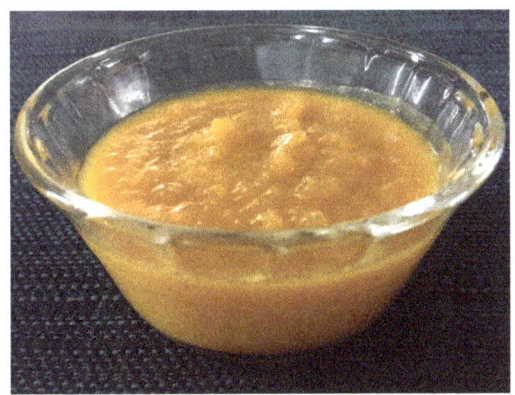

Heat the butter and cook the onion until soft for 5–10 minutes. Peel, deseed, and cut butternut squash into cubes. Add broth, squash, ginger (optional, if so grate it), and cumin and cook about 20 minutes on medium heat. Puree in blender when squash is cooked. In a separate pan, bring the water and quinoa to a boil, reduce heat to low, cover, and simmer until quinoa is tender and water is absorbed after 15–20 minutes. Add quinoa to soup bowls and serve.

I have used carnival and acorn squash for this recipe, and both are just as delicious as the butternut squash.

Since it is a vegetarian soup, I prefer vegetable broth for this recipe.

If you do not want to add the quinoa, you don't have to, it makes a great creamy soup as it is.

Lentil, Kale, and Potato Soup

1 tbsp. olive oil
1 medium onion, diced
2 stalks celery, diced
2 large carrots, diced
1 cup dry lentils, rinsed
4 cups vegetable broth
1/2 cup water
1/2 tsp. garlic powder
1/4 tsp. cumin
1 large potato, diced
1/2 bunch Kale, ribs removed
pepper to taste

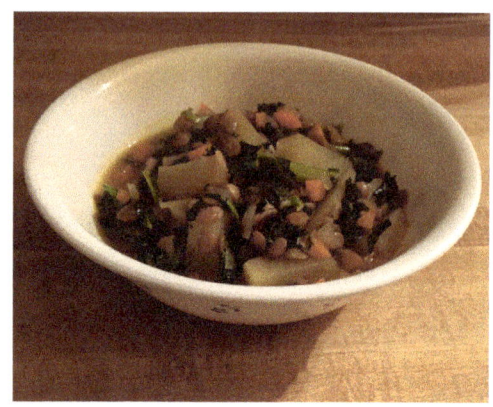

Heat olive oil in a large pot over medium heat. Add onion, celery, and carrots and sauté until softened, about 10 minutes.

Add lentils, broth, water, garlic, and cumin. Stir together and bring to a boil. Once soup has reached a boil, reduce heat to low and simmer, cover for 20 minutes. Add chopped potatoes and simmer, cover for 15 more minutes or until potatoes are fork tender. Add kale and simmer, cover for an additional 5 minutes, or until kale is wilted. Remove from heat and season with pepper.

When kale is not in season, I have used 1/2 bag of frozen chopped kale. Also, do not use red lentils in this soup, I use organic sprouted green lentils. You can use 1/4 tsp. coriander in this recipe, and I sometimes add 1/4 tsp. extra of cumin, up to you!

Potato Leek Soup

3 large leeks, finely chopped
2 lbs. potatoes, diced
4 cups vegetable broth
1 tsp. Italian spices
1/2 tsp. black pepper to taste
1 tbsp. butter

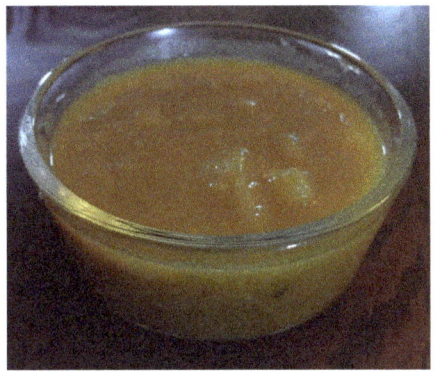

Clean leeks, cut dark tough green tops off and discard. Slice white and green part in half and then cut crosswise 1/4" thick. Dice potatoes smaller for less cooking time. Melt butter and on medium heat, add leeks and cook for 10 minutes until softened but not brown. Increase heat to high and add potatoes and broth, cook till it simmers then reduce the heat to low and cook 20 minutes or until the potatoes are cooked through. Once it is cooked through, puree soup in a blender but leave some leeks and potatoes whole. Add puree back to the pieces you reserved and add pepper to taste.

You can use either an immersion or standing blender.

Yukon and yellow potatoes both work fine in this recipe. I also use fresh fennel in this recipe for some added flavor, finely chop them the same as your leeks.

Smoked Turkey Soup

1 yellow onion, finely chopped
4 celery stalks, finely chopped
20–24 baby carrots, chopped
3 cloves garlic, minced
1 roasted red pepper, chopped
1 1/2 cups smoked organic turkey
pre-cooked and chopped
1 cup wild rice
1 32 oz. organic chicken broth
extra 16 oz. chicken broth
1/3 cup flour
2 3/4 cup almond milk
1/4 tsp. black pepper

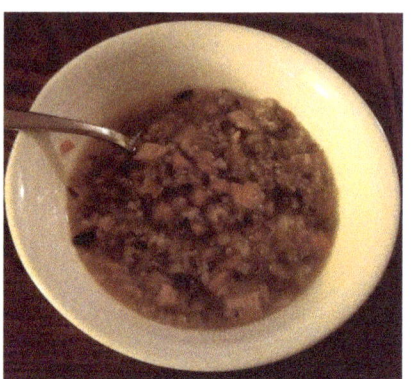

Cook rice with 16 oz. of chicken broth. Prep all the ingredients while the rice is cooking. Rice will be cooked by the time you need to add it to the soup. Cooking it in the broth will help the soup to add a bit of thickness. In the stockpot, add veggies and sauté. Slowly add chicken broth and stir in turkey and rice. Bring to a boil, once boiling reduce heat to medium and add the chopped roasted red pepper. Simmer. Meanwhile, whisk the milk and flour together and let stand to get to room temperature. Add to the pot and stir constantly till it is folded in. Cook over medium heat to thicken for 10-15 minutes longer.

The last step with the flour and milk can be omitted if you do not want a thicker soup. I have done them both ways but now I have opted to not use this mixture. Also, this soup is best with a real on the bone turkey. I always make this soup in the days following Thanksgiving with our turkey leftovers.

Tomato Basil Soup

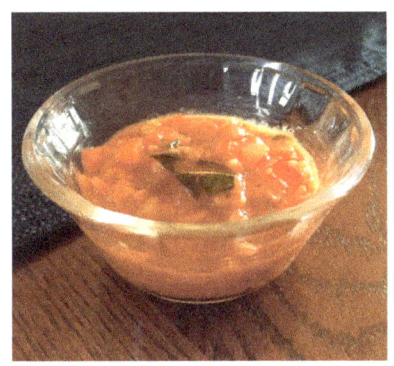

3 carrots, peeled and diced fine
1/2 onion, chopped fine
1/2 red pepper, diced fine
3 celery stalks, diced fine
1 clove garlic, minced
2 28 oz. cans crushed tomatoes with herbs
1 carton 32 oz. vegetable stock
2 roasted red peppers, diced
1 cup orzo pasta or 1/2 cup rice
1 cup almond milk or light cream
2 tbsp. fresh basil, chopped

Add vegetables and garlic to your stockpot and heat on medium low for 5 minutes until tender, stir often so it doesn't stick or burn. Add the tomatoes and simmer for about 10 minutes. Now add your stock and return to a simmer, cover for about 10 minutes or so. Season with pepper and add red peppers and pasta, simmer for about 10–20 minutes stirring often until the pasta or rice is firm but tender. Remove from heat.

Temper cream. Pour cream into medium bowl, add a few ladles of hot soup to the cream to slowly raise the cream temperature.

Add this cream mixture to the soup and fold in the basil.

Momma's Organic Vegetable Soup

1/2 10 oz. bag broccoli, frozen
1 10 oz. bag mixed vegetables, frozen
1 14.5 oz. diced tomatoes with herbs
1 15 oz. can garbanzo beans
1 32 oz. carton vegetable broth

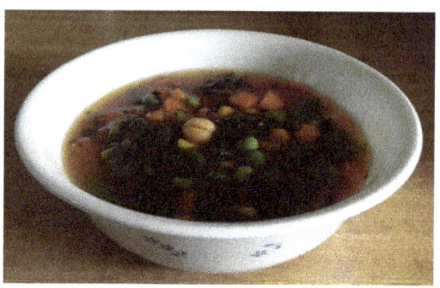

Mix all ingredients and cook for 20-30 minutes.

Super easy! If you eat pasta you can add that or tortellini, my family usually just tops it with a little bit of Romano cheese.

In the summer I use the fresh vegetables from my farm share, it may take a little longer to cook but it is worth the fresh flavors!

In the winter I always use whatever vegetables I may have frozen from my summer share or I buy organic frozen vegetables.

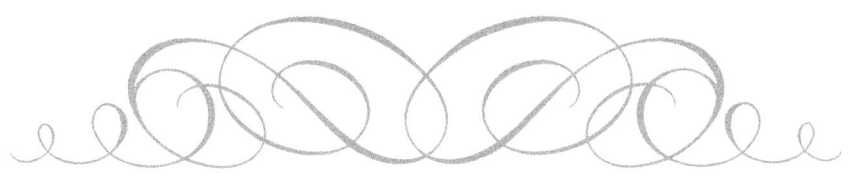

Salads

Jesus said to them, "I am the bread of life, whoever comes to me will never hunger, and whoever believes in me will never thirst."

—John 6:35

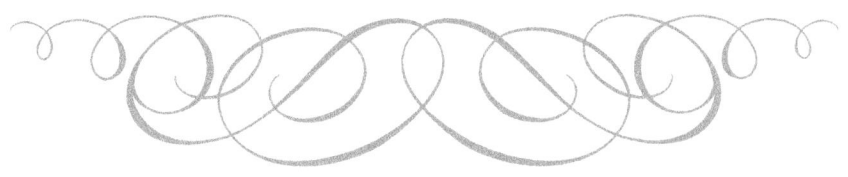

I have been told in the past, "If there was a simple guide I would just follow it, why does it have to be so hard?" Well, it doesn't have to be so hard. You do need to be dedicated to your health though, and keep a few things in mind whenever tempting foods cross your path. So here is my simple guide I always tell myself, stay away from any and all processed foods, lower your sugar intake daily, lower your red meats, and when eating animal products, pay attention to where the animals are from and the farming practices. Labeling is not regulated so some things can say something but not actually practice it, try to eat wild and grass fed, drink water and not juices, sugary drinks, or alcohol, and finally, eat a rainbow of organic fruits and vegetables.

Simple and obvious, right?

Well, not always easy to follow and too easy sometimes to say, well, only once in a while, yes, in moderation, can be okay but then sometimes we fall into moderation more often and it no longer is in moderation. I know it sounds crazy but if I see something tempting, I tend to look at it more as to how it was made in a factory I stay away from completely! And add a salad or two daily, this truly does help you stay on your nutritional track.

There is so many ways to serve a salad, you can be as creative or boring, it really doesn't matter. Kind of anything goes, but with my family, I have to be very creative. If they had their choice they would not opt for a salad, I am sure you can all relate or may feel the same way my family does. When I make salads they can easily be converted into wraps, if you are the person that needs a carb wrapped around your salad. The perfect salad would consist of many different kinds of vegetables, combined with a protein and a healthy fat.

You will notice a few of my recipes are pasta based, okay, I am Italian, so pasta has been a staple in my diet most of my life. When I was younger, I think it is all I ate, especially when I started life on my own. It is the cheapest meal you can ever make, and maybe this is why, because it has next to no nutritional value. Our wheat industry is not like your great grandparents' generation and definitely not of Jesus's time. We can eat wheat in the US but it wrecks havoc on every human being and animal's digestive system. Our bodies were made to repair themselves, and they can, but only for so long before it is too late and you are diagnosed with some sort of degenerative disease.

Why is this, you may ask, well, it used to be that when wheat was grown it was grown to its full potential of over four feet tall, but now modern wheat or dwarf wheat stands just two feet high and has been crossbred to cultivate an abnormally large seed head balanced on a stocky stem. There are a lot of factors that come into play—how wheat was grown, cultivated, processed, etc. All of which now seem to be causing it to have less nutrients, more carbohydrates, and higher amounts of phytic acid, which reduces the absorption of calcium, magnesium, iron, copper, and zinc.

I have chosen for my family to stay away from it as best we can, including my dog. Actually, my dog does a better job at it than we do because she doesn't have the choice as to what we feed her.

It is strange for me to not make as many pasta dishes as I once did, but I have seen the effects on all of us and until I figure out a better way, I chose to make pasta dishes on occasion. For now, I have been purchasing rice pasta or a bean based pasta that has three ingredients, nothing foreign, and has no gluten naturally. Surprisingly, for the dishes I make it with, you really can't taste the difference. The only thing is you are limited to the types of pasta, so as of now I don't make my lasagna, I make what I call a lazy lasagna and I can't make my manicotti, which is to die for, just saying! Oh, I can't forget about my stuffed shells, okay, the Italian momma is coming out with all the amazing food I haven't been able to make, but one day, in the near future, I will figure out how to make my own pasta that won't hurt you in the end.

I think you will agree my favorite salads offer so many great flavors you may forget you are eating a salad and I don't think you will miss the wheat in my pasta salad dishes.

Avocado Salad

1 whole avocado, diced
baby romaine or mixed salad greens
1 carrot, diced
1 tomato, diced
1/2 cucumber, diced
1 pepper, diced
1/4 red onion, diced
1/2 can garbanzo beans

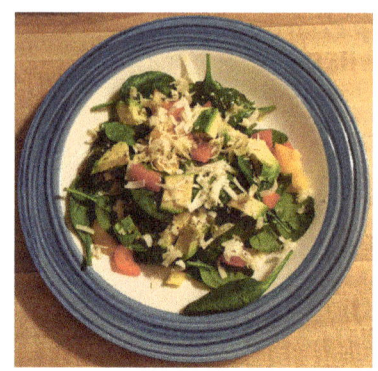

    This is my go-to salad during the week, we have this salad once a week and I change it up a bit. If I am going to put cheese on it, organic white cheddar is what pair perfectly with this salad, and then we do not have dressing. If we have dressing, it is always my homemade Greek dressing or my Vinaigrette because I do not buy bottled dressings any longer.

    This salad feeds my family of three and sometimes I make a little more so we have this for our lunches the following day.

    I use about 1 cup each of greens per salad.

Avocado, Artichoke Chopped Salad

3 cups raw spinach, chopped
1/2 avocado, chopped
4 artichoke hearts, diced
8 grape tomatoes, diced
6 baby carrots, diced
1 cup broccoli florets
1/2 can garbanzo beans, drained
1/4 cup blue cheese crumbles
1/4 cup black olives, sliced

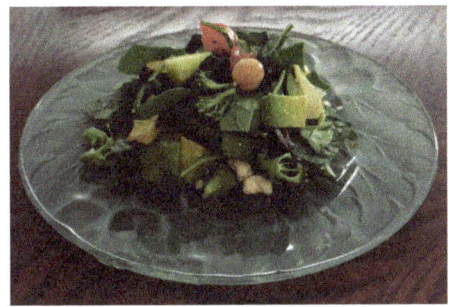

Chop and dice all ingredients and add to a large bowl. Once everything is prepared add the blue cheese crumbles and give it a good mix, so when you serve, everyone gets all of the ingredients.

If you have a chopper, hand chop all ingredients, it gives off a very fresh taste. I don't have one and tend to do everything by hand, so a knife will do the trick too!

Beet Avocado Salad

1/2 small garlic clove
1 tbsp. lemon juice
2 tbsp. olive oil
1/2 avocado, chopped
2 small beets, diced
2 cups baby romaine

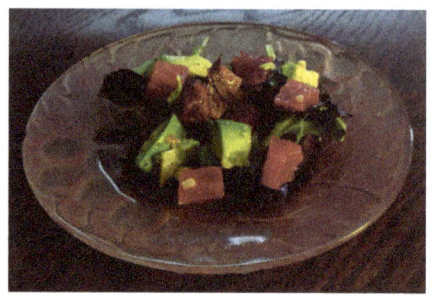

Dressing:
    Finely chop or mince the garlic, if you do not have a mincer you can finely chop and with a back of a spoon, smash against the bowl until almost pasty. Mix garlic with olive oil and lemon juice and whisk well. Set aside.
    In a serving bowl, place the baby romaine, beets, and avocado. Pour prepared dressing over the top, if it separated whisk again.
    Arugula works well with this salad also.
    You can use roasted beets or steamed beets in this recipe.

Buffalo Chicken Salad

3 chicken breasts, cooked
12 dashes hot sauce
3 cups romaine
1 tomato, diced
2–3 celery stalks, diced
10 baby carrots, diced
1/4 cup blue cheese crumbles

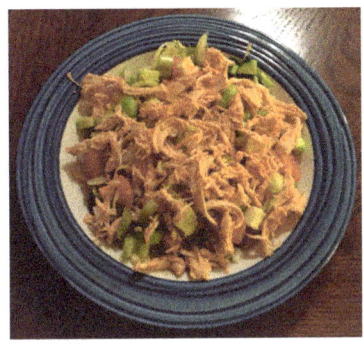

Cook chicken thoroughly, heat olive oil and add raw chicken cubed, or you can boil the chicken and shred it, both ways are good. Make sure the internal temperature is 165 degrees. Once the chicken is thoroughly cooked, mix with the hot sauce over low heat.

Add layers of each ingredient on top of 1 cup of the romaine salad. I evenly distribute each ingredient.

I use Frank's hot sauce, this makes it a true buffalo chicken salad!

I use Baby Romaine or Super Greens for this salad. I also sometimes add avocado slices to this salad.

Brussels Sprout Slaw

1 pkg. brussels sprouts, shredded
1 red pepper, diced
1/2 cup raw almonds, chopped
1/2 bunch green onions, thinly sliced
3/4 cup Momma's Vinaigrette
pepper to taste

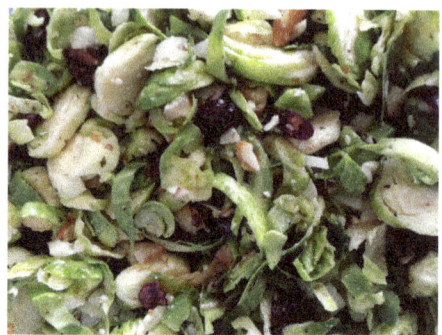

Chop everything, your brussels sprouts should be about 14 oz., you can buy them preshredded or finely chop yourself. The red pepper should be about 1 cup, I have a chopper to chop my almonds or you can chop them in a food processor. Mix everything together and add the vinaigrette and the pepper. Put lid on your container and toss to coat.

Chill a half hour or overnight. This can be served by itself, as a side to a meal, or added to a salad.

Guac Lentil Salad

3 cups water
1 cup lentils
1 can fire roasted tomatoes
1 avocado
1 tbsp. lemon juice
3 cups romaine lettuce

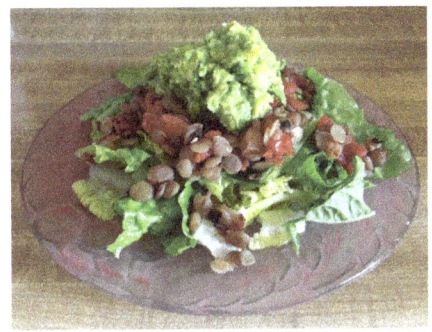

Prepare lentils according to package directions with the water and lentils. Make Guacamole according to my recipe. Chop romaine lettuce while the lentils are cooking and prepare your guacamole.

After your lentils are cooked, you may need to drain some extra water. Now add the fire-roasted tomatoes and heat a few extra minutes. Once lentils have cooled slightly top each salad. I use about a cup for each plate of the romaine. And now add your guacamole to top it off.

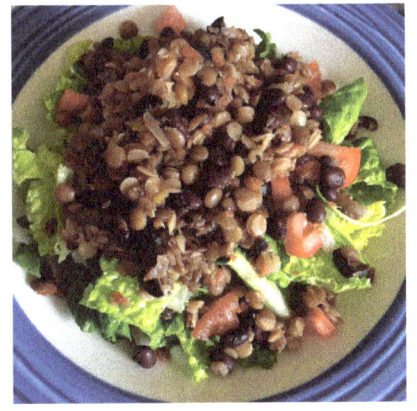

I have used crushed and diced tomatoes in this recipe, the picture is shown with diced.

If you do not want guacamole you can use the lentils and black beans.

Hummus Salad

raw spinach
1 15.5 oz. garbanzo beans, drained
1 carrot, diced
1/2 cucumber, diced
1/4 red onion, diced
hummus

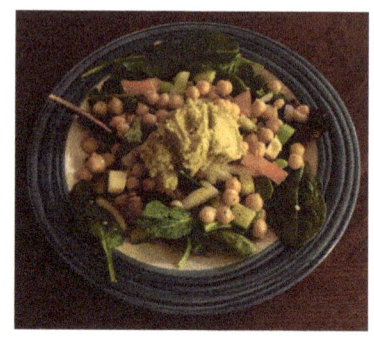

I use the hummus I have made for the week, Avocado hummus, Beet Hummus, Garlic Hummus, and Red Pepper Hummus all of them work wonderful!

I use 2 tsp. per salad of hummus. I use about 1/4 cup garbanzo beans per salad. My veggies change individually, I love onions but my daughter doesn't so I may use tomatoes on hers instead.

If you need measuring, try to use under 1/4 cup for each of your veggies and about 1 cup per salad of your raw spinach. If this is our main meal, everyone will get 1 1/2–2 cups veggies per serving.

Make extras for lunches tomorrow!

Kohlrabi Salad

A small kohlrabi, 1 cup
A small cabbage, 5 cups
4 carrots
Vinaigrette

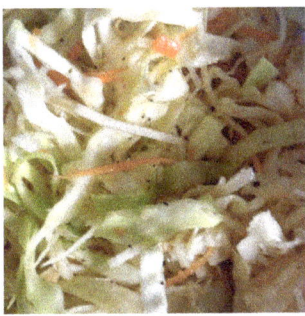

Cut cabbage in four and core, slice and add to a large bowl. Trim kohlrabi and shred fine on a mandolin. Add kohlrabi to the cabbage and mix in 1/2 the vinaigrette. Continue shredding the kohlrabi and chopping the cabbage and carrots. Now add the remainder of the vinaigrette and mix well. You can serve right away or chill in the refrigerator.

You will use all of the vinaigrette in this recipe. You can use green or purple cabbage, but I prefer the green.

Lemon, Garbanzo, Tuna Salad

2 15.5 oz. cans garbanzo beans, rinsed
2–3 Roma tomatoes, chopped
1/2 red onion, finely chopped
1 bunch flat leaf parsley, finely chopped
1/2 bunch mint, finely chopped
1/2 tsp. lemon zest
3 tbsp. lemon juice
1 tbsp. olive oil
1 clove garlic, minced
2 5 oz. cans wild tuna in natural juices, mixed not drained

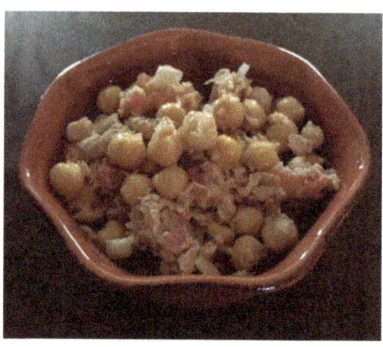

Mix herbs, lemon juice, olive oil, and garlic together then pour over the beans, tomatoes and onion. Fold in the tuna last.

You can also add finely chopped cucumber to this, and when I make this in the winter and the herbs are not fresh, I have omitted them and it has come out wonderful also. This is a family favorite!

It can be served alone, on a bed of mixed greens, or served as an appetizer with pita slices.

Potato Salad

5 lbs. baby red potatoes
2 5 oz. plain Greek yogurts
6 scallions, diced
2 tsp. black pepper

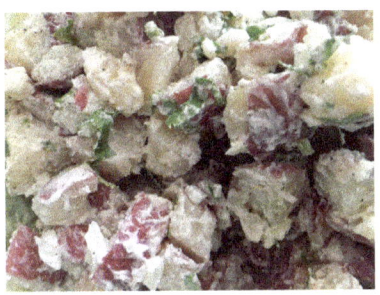

    Wash and dice the potatoes, add them to a large stockpot full of cold water. Once all the potatoes are cut and added to your pot, cook them on medium heat for 20–30 minutes or until the potatoes are tender. Drain them in a colander and let cool for a 1/2 an hour to 45 minutes.

    Meanwhile, dice the scallions or green onions, whichever both work great. Trim the tops and the bottoms. I use some of the greens, about 3–4 inches of the whole stalk of the onion.

    Once the potatoes are cooled, transfer them to your container to mix with the yogurt, scallions or green onions and black pepper.

    Once combined refrigerate overnight. If before serving it is not as creamy as you would like, add 1/4–1/2 of another container of plain Greek yogurt.

Tuna Noodle Salad

1 pkg. spiral rice pasta
2 cans wild Albacore tuna
2 celery stalks, diced
1/2 cup peas, frozen
1/4 cup onion, diced
20 pickles, diced
1 tsp. black pepper
2–5 oz. plain Greek yogurt

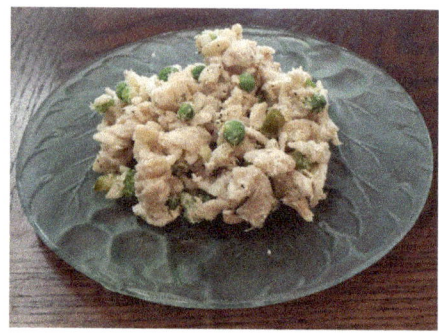

Cook pasta according to directions. Meanwhile, chop all of the vegetable ingredients.

Do not drain the tuna, if you buy the kind I do, it is in its natural juices and this is important for us to eat. Blend it together with a fork.

Once the pasta is cooked and drained you will fold the tuna into the pasta and add 1 container of the yogurt. Mix together and start to add the vegetables.

If you are serving this salad the next day or later in the day stop here; prior to serving add the second container of yogurt and the pepper.

If you think it may still be too dry, add a little extra yogurt but this comes out perfect for my family.

Vegetable Pasta Salad

1 box rotini, cooked
5 oz. broccoli florets, small
10 grape tomatoes, cut
12 olives, cut in 3rds
1/2 cup red pepper, diced
4 oz. X-Sharp cheddar, cubed
4 oz. mozzarella or Romano, cubed
vinaigrette

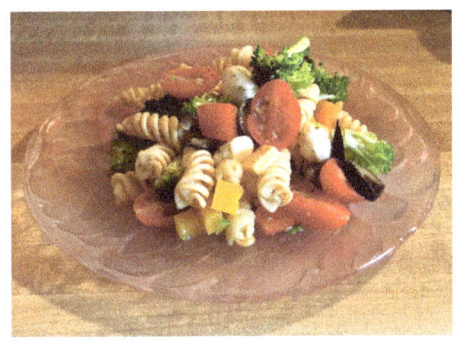

Cook pasta according to their directions, once cooked and drained, rinse under cold water and drain again.

Add chopped vegetables, vegetables may vary to your taste and if you think you want more vegetables please add more!

Add vinaigrette and mix well, do this one more time to taste about 1/4–1/2 cup vinaigrette.

If you refrigerate this salad you may need to add more vinaigrette before serving as it soaks into the pasta.

The pasta I tend to use is a rice based pasta but in the picture above I used a chickpea pasta and it turned out fantastic!

When making this recipe with my vinaigrette, you will make 2 batches of the vinaigrette and mix well. Refrigerate and taste and add one more batch of the vinaigrette for best results!

Watermelon Salad

Salad

2 large tomatoes, cut (2 cups)
2 lbs. watermelon, cut 1/2"x1/2" wedges
1 cucumber, peeled and cut 1/2" wedges
1/2 small red onion, thinly sliced (1/4 cup)

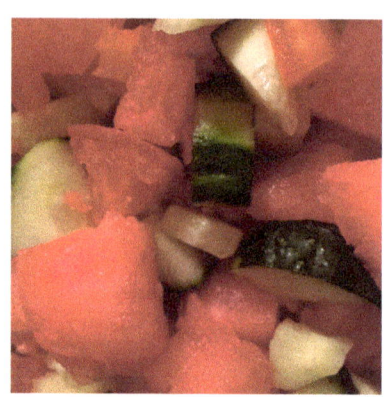

Dressing

3 tbsps. apple cider vinegar or red wine vinegar
2 tbsps. extra virgin olive oil
1/4 tsp. pepper
1/4 cup fresh basil leaves, sliced

Once cut gently toss everything together with the dressing, refrigerate up to 2 hours and sprinkle with basil.

I love this salad in the summertime, it is so light and refreshing, your family will love it! Mine does!

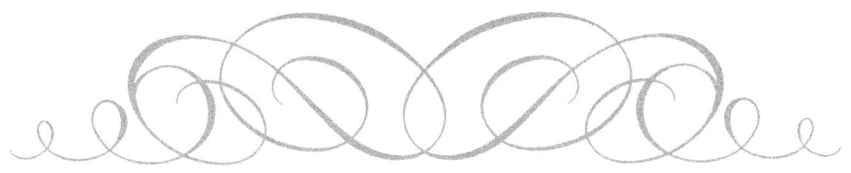

Sides

For I am the *Lord*, your *God*, who grasp your right hand; it is I who say to you, "Fear not, *I will help you*."

—Isaiah 41:13

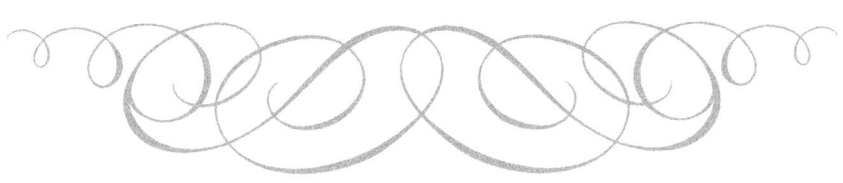

The American plate usually consists of a vegetable, a starch, and a protein. I think you would agree most meals have a side added or two. My meals rarely have a side but that doesn't mean I don't make them. It really depends on the meal. Some of my meals are only accompanied by a small salad and some of my meals are just what they are because of everything created inside of it.

But even when I think of my main dishes, I still start them with a small salad, so if you are not in the mood for a salad these may be easy additions you can refer to and serve with your meal.

I tried to think of my family's favorites, some I make more often than others and I am sure you will be able to figure out which ones are the ones we tend to. Nothing will take you too long to prepare and you will be able to prepare them while your main dishes are cooking.

This was always a struggle for me—to time my meals properly—but over time I have gotten this down and am able to serve everything warm and ready to eat.

So, on those occasions, I do make a side to go with a meal, these are the sides I tend to make. I hope you enjoy them as much as my family and friends do!

Baked Beans

1 lg sweet onion, diced
3 tbsp. butter
1/2 cup maple syrup
1/3 cup lemon juice
2 tbsp. brown sugar
2 tbsp. tomato paste
1/2 tsp. pepper
2 15 oz. cans pinto beans
2 15 oz. cans cannellini beans
1 15 oz. can garbanzo beans

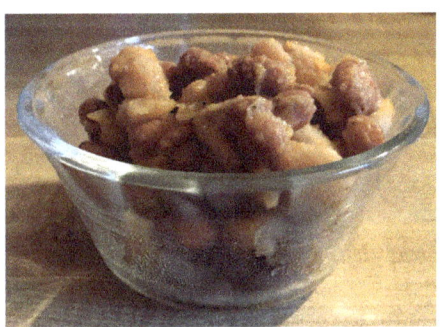

Drain all the beans, and chop and dice the onion. Heat the butter on medium heat, once the butter is melted, add the diced onion and cook until the onion is a bit translucent. Add the maple syrup, lemon juice, brown sugar, tomato paste, and pepper. Stir all the ingredients together, once they are combined you can add the beans. After adding each can of beans mix the pot really well to coat. Now reduce your heat to simmer and cover, cook for 15–20 minutes.

When purchasing a maple syrup, a dark grade is preferred when cooking.

This will be a hearty baked bean recipe, if you like it with more liquid then you can reduce the amount of beans you add. But my family prefers it this way.

I sometimes lower the maple syrup to 1/4 cup and no one can tell the difference, if you would like to cut back on the sugar I suggest doing this.

Buffalo Cauliflower

1 head cauliflower
1/2 cup garbanzo bean flour
1/2 cup water
1 tsp. garlic powder
1 tsp. butter, melted
2/3 cup Frank's hot sauce

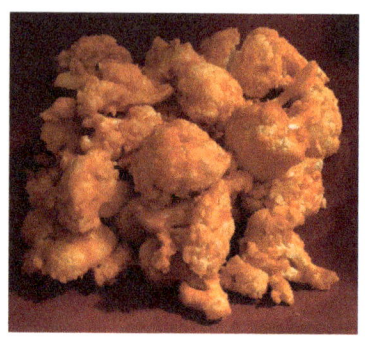

Preheat oven to 450 degrees. Chop cauliflower into bite-sized pieces and add them to a medium-sized bowl. Combine flour, garlic powder, and water, whisk together until smooth.

Toss the cauliflower with the batter, making sure to coat all the pieces. Place the battered cauliflower on the preheated pizza stone, or a lightly greased cookie sheet. Bake for 15 minutes, flipping halfway through.

In a large bowl combine the melted butter and Frank's hot sauce and stir together. When cauliflower is done, remove from the oven and toss it with your hot sauce mix. Place cauliflower, bake on the pan you were using and bake another 25 minutes until the cauliflower becomes crispy. Cool before serving.

I use Frank's hot sauce because it is the best, if you do not have Frank's you can use whatever hot sauce you prefer.

Easy Buffalo Cauliflower

1 head cauliflower
1/2 cup Frank's hot sauce

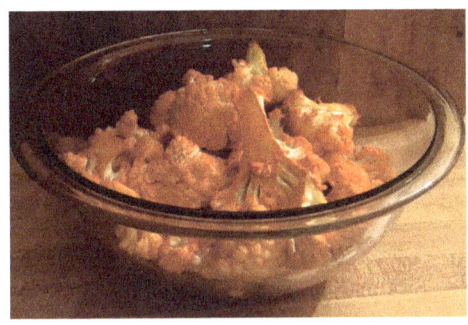

Preheat oven to 400 degrees, and bake stone for at least 20 minutes. Wash and cut cauliflower into florets then mix together with the hot sauce.

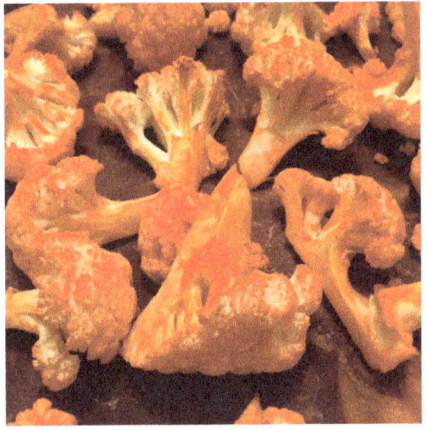

Place cauliflower on pizza stone and bake 45 minutes turning once in between. Some water will come out of the cauliflower but with the hot pizza stone, it will easily evaporate.

Garlic Kale

1 tbsp. olive oil
2 cloves garlic, chopped
6 cups kale, fresh

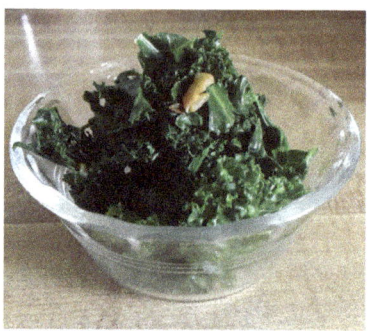

On medium heat, heat oil and add chopped garlic. Sauté a few minutes to brown but not burn, add 3 cups of the destemmed kale and mix constantly with the garlic. As it cooks down add 1 cup at a time the rest of the kale until all 6 cups are in your pan. This will be about a 5-minute cook time till all the kale is added, now turn off heat and cover till serving.

If you do not have kale, Swiss chard or collard greens I cook the same way.

Mashed Potatoes

6–7 potatoes, 2 lbs.
1 carton chicken broth, 4 cups

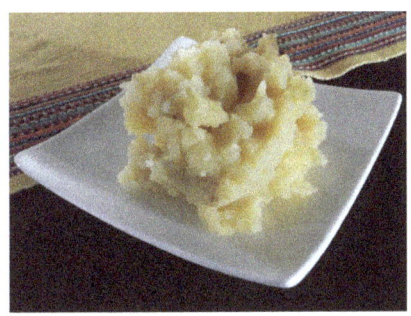

Dice the potatoes and bring chicken broth and potatoes to a boil. Boil for about 25 minutes.

Drain broth but reserve it in case the potatoes need a little extra liquid. Season with pepper if you would like and serve warm.

Mashed Sweet Potatoes with Cheddar

3 lbs. sweet potatoes
1 1/2 cups XX sharp cheddar
water to boil

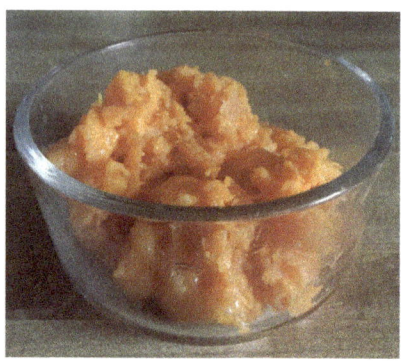

    Peel and dice the potatoes into small pieces. Add them to your pot of water and do not turn the stove on until all the potatoes are added. You will boil them on medium heat about 20 minutes until they are fully cooked.

    Drain and Mash the potatoes, add the shredded cheddar, and mash again. You will see they will become creamier once the cheese is blended into the potatoes.

    This is a great way to get your family to love sweet potatoes, they are the best potato and are a great source of vitamin A, vitamin B6, and potassium. My family is not the biggest fan but love it when I make them this way!

    I use the sharpest cheddar I can find so the taste does come through in this recipe.

Roasted Asparagus

1 bunch asparagus
  or
1 pkg. frozen asparagus
1/4 cup Pecorino Romano

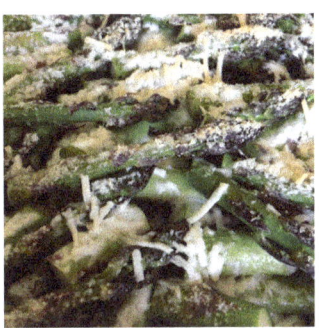

Chop asparagus in half and place in a Pyrex pan, top with Pecorino Romano cheese and roast on 450 degrees about 10 minutes or until tender and cheese is starting to melt.

Roasted Asparagus with Garlic

1 lb. fresh asparagus
2 tsp. olive oil
2 garlic cloves, minced
pepper to taste

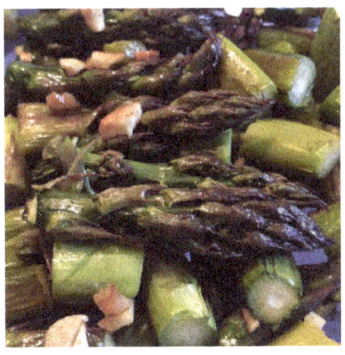

Preheat oven to 500 degrees.
In Pyrex shallow pie pan place asparagus and coat with olive oil. Sprinkle garlic and pepper to taste. Roast uncovered for 6–8 minutes shaking pan occasionally.
I like garlic, so for mine I added 5 cloves chopped garlic. It is not overpowering but so good!

Roasted Beets

2–8 beets
olive oil

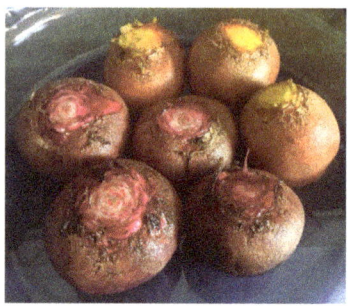

    Preheat oven to 375 degrees, remove the stem and most of the root from your beets, and scrub and wash them under water until clean.

    Place your beets in a Pyrex glass baking dish. Drizzle with a little olive oil and roast for an hour or until a knife inserted falls out without resistance. They should be tender. You can set them in the fridge to cool to room temperature if using in a recipe right away.

Steamed Beets

    Trim beets, like above and then steam whole over boiling water until tender when pierced with a fork, but not too soft. A medium size beet can take about 25 minutes. I usually make 4 at a time. When done, cool and then trim the skin. Cut beets into wedges or large diced pieces.

Roasted Broccoli

1 head broccoli
  or
1 pkg. frozen broccoli
1/4 cup Pecorino Romano,
  shredded

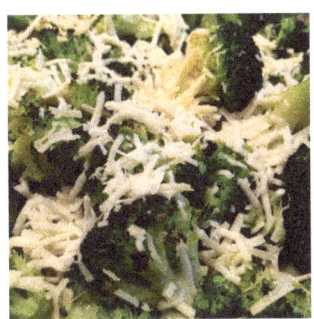

If using fresh broccoli, rinse well and chop into florets. Place broccoli in Pyrex pan and top with Pecorino Romano. Roast on 450 degrees for about 15 minutes.

Roasted Cauliflower

1 head cauliflower
 or
1 pkg. frozen cauliflower
1/4 cup Pecorino Romano,
  shredded

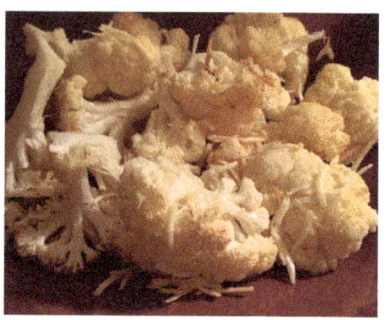

    If using fresh cauliflower, rinse well and chop into florets.
    Place cauliflower in Pyrex pan and top with Pecorino Romano. Roast on 450 degrees about 15 minutes.

Roasted Spaghetti Squash

1 spaghetti squash cut in 1/2, deseeded
olive oil

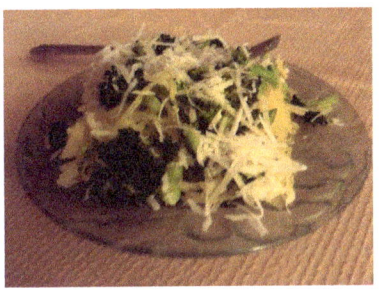

Preheat oven to 375 degrees.

Cut spaghetti squash in 1/2 and deseed, rub the inside with olive oil and on a non-stick pan place it upside down.

Bake approximately 35–45 minutes and let stand 5 minutes before using a fork and get strands out of the shell.

Serve with Momma's Sauce or roasted vegetables and shredded Romano cheese.

Scalloped Potatoes

7 potatoes (about 2 pounds)
1 onion
1 1/2 cups almond milk
1 8 oz. brick x-sharp cheddar
1/4 tsp. black pepper

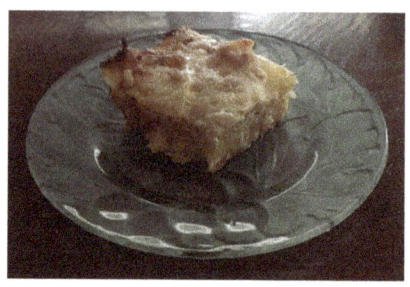

Preheat oven at 400 degrees and prepare a glass baking pan with coconut oil. With a mandolin, slice potatoes, dice onion, and shred cheddar.

You will start layering with your potatoes, then onion, and finally the cheese. On the 3rd layer add the pepper. Once all of your ingredients are used, pour the almond milk all over the scalloped potatoes.

Bake for 45 minutes and add another layer of cheese to the top, return to oven for 10-15 minutes until melted.

I have used many different potatoes in this recipe but I do like the yellow potatoes best.

If the skins look good and you do not have any brown spots or sprouting on your potatoes do not peel them. If you need to peel them that is okay, it will come out great any way you make them!

Stuffing

2 loaves bakery bread, diced
1 yellow onion, medium
1 cup celery
1/2–3/4 cup carrots
32 oz. chicken broth
1 1/2 tbsp. Italian seasonings
1 tbsp. pepper

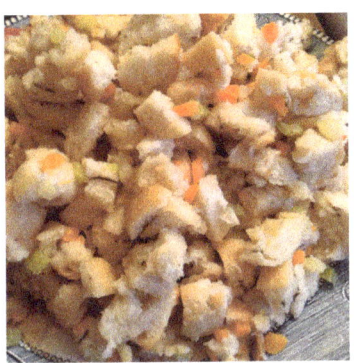

Dice bread the night before serving and leave on a cookie sheet in the oven to get a bit crusty.

Finely dice all vegetables and cook in the broth for a half an hour. When it boils add to the bread in an olive oiled lasagna pan. While stirring add Italian seasonings and pepper. If the mixture is not completely wet, add more broth and vegetables.

Bake at 350 degrees for an hour. Check often and add broth and veggies if need be.

I make this stuffing at Thanksgiving, and because I want it to cook at the same time as my turkey I cook extra broth and celery if I will need it.

This year I cooked it at the same time as my turkey and scalloped potatoes so I baked everything at 450 degrees for a half an hour and everything turned out perfect!

Zucchini Marinara

2 zucchini
1 onion
2 tomatoes

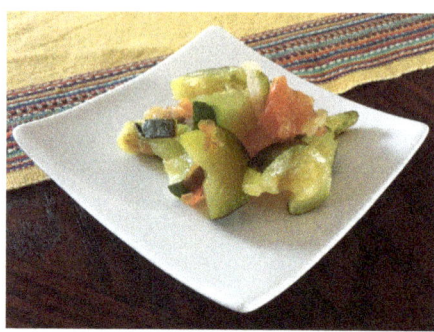

    Slice all vegetables and add to your pan. The zucchini will create its own juice so there is no need for olive oil, but it adds flavor and nutrition if you add 1 teaspoon.

    Cover and let steam for 15 minutes, stirring every 5 minutes. Once vegetables are softened, in 15–20 minutes they are ready to be served.

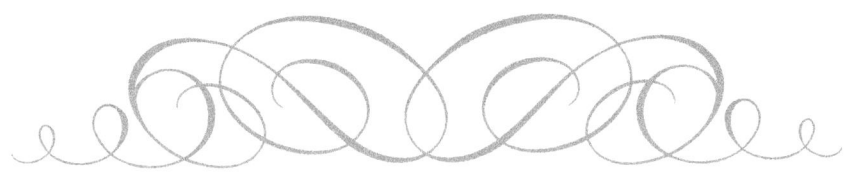

Sandwiches

Jesus said in reply, "It is written: One does not live by *Bread* alone, but by every *Word* that comes forth from the mouth of *God*."

—Matthew 4:4

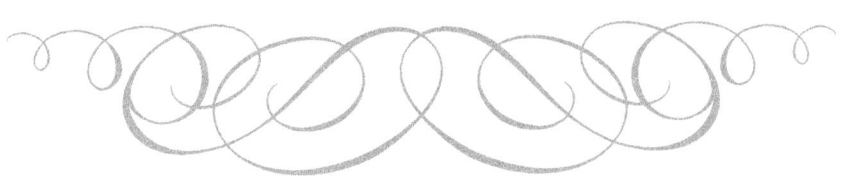

Now that I have touched on my issue with wheat, I am sure you probably think my family does not eat sandwiches. Sandwiches technically are improperly combined foods, protein and starches don't mix well in our digestive system. Starches and proteins are considered concentrated foods, food that does not contain water. For maximum digestion we should eat 1 concentrated food at a time, and technically you should wait 3–4 hours in between them so we have time to clear the first food out of our stomach.

Now I am just touching on a few facts and won't bore you with the movement of our digestive track, but from this little bit you can see where a sandwich is not a good idea, but we have all been raised on sandwiches. And I think we can all agree they taste delicious. But food that tastes delicious isn't always good for us.

So, my answer is yes, every once in a while, my family does eat sandwiches, and even though I know we will not get the optimal nutrition we should get from that sandwich, I prepare our day a little different.

How?

By having an incredibly healthy salad for lunch and then the sandwich, which is also served with a salad for dinner. And remember what I told you, it could become a habit for everyone to eat their salads before their sandwiches, and if you want to take it a step further serve your salads before you have finished making the sandwiches so your bodies have that rest time in between to digest.

You will notice some of my sandwiches do not include animal protein, they will include protein from either beans or avocados. Also, some of these recipes you can skip the bread all together, it is truly up to you. I will do that a lot of times and make it into a salad, where my family will prefer the sandwich!

Now speaking of bread, always choose organic if possible, sour dough is best, and read labels! Stay away from canola and soybean oil, neither should be in bread, if any oil is, it should be olive. And added gluten is not needed to make bread, if I see that on the label, I skip it. Your best bet is five ingredients or less. One day I will find the time to perfect my own, that day hasn't come yet but stay tuned because it could be.

In the pages that follow you will see my family's favorite sandwiches that I make, I hope you enjoy them as much as they do!

Avocado Vegetable Panini

6 slices organic bread
1 avocado
8–10 grape tomatoes
1/2 pepper, sliced
1 cup raw spinach
1 cup x-sharp cheddar
1/4 of an onion

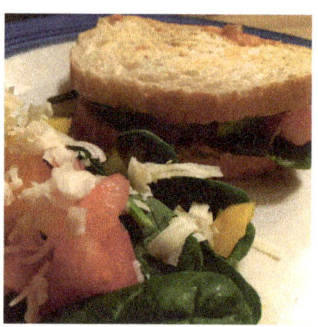

This is a sandwich you can change all the time, as I have said in the past, I am a fan of onion where my family not so much so when I use it I slice the onion thinly and only add it to some sandwiches.

I love to use the organic rosemary bread but the organic sourdough is really good too!

You will layer the sandwiches with the shredded cheese then the spinach around 5–6 leaves. The tomatoes I slice in 4 and add them now so they stack and stay on the sandwich. Slice the peppers like the onions and add them to the top before another thin layer of cheese.

I make 3 sandwiches at a time on my pan and use a smaller lid to push them down to make them into a panini. Five minutes on each side till golden brown and they are ready to serve. This will make 6 sandwiches.

Black Bean Burger

2 cloves garlic, minced
4 cups black beans, cooked
1 tsp. ground cumin
1 cup panko bread crumbs
1 egg, beaten
1 tbsp. coconut oil

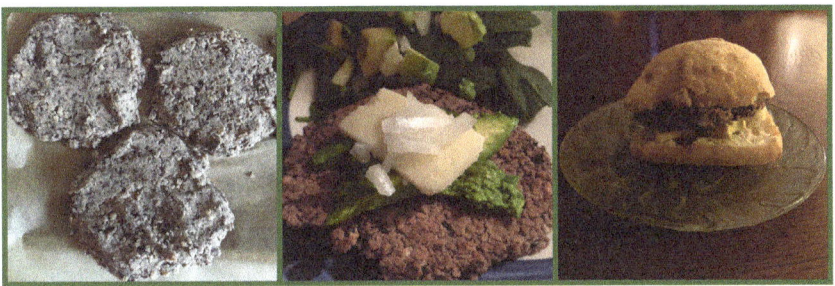

In a food processor blend garlic, black beans, panko, cumin, and egg. Blend well.

Use a tablespoon and scoop out mix, place on parchment paper on a baking sheet and form patties, they will be about 3" round each.

In a pan melt coconut oil for 2 minutes then add 2–4 patties depending on the size of your pan. Fry about 5 minutes on each side over medium high heat until brown.

I make 10 out of this mixture.

You can make sandwiches and top with avocado slices and cheddar, or go bunless and serve with a salad.

Buffalo Chicken Salad Wrap

3 chicken breasts, cooked
12 dashes hot sauce
3 cups romaine
1 tomato, diced
2–3 celery stalks, diced
10 baby carrots, diced
1/4 cup blue cheese crumbles
3 lavash or pita flat breads

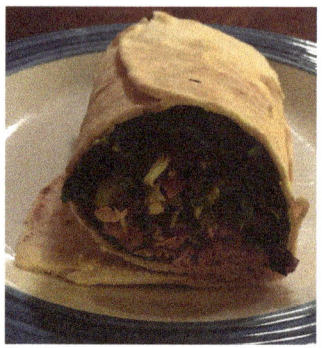

Cook chicken thoroughly, heat olive oil, and add raw chicken cubed, or you can boil the chicken and shred it, both ways are good. Make sure the internal temperature is 165 degrees. Once the chicken is thoroughly cooked, mix with the hot sauce over low heat.

Add layers of each topping to the lavash or pita flat bread. I evenly distribute each ingredient and then wrap the sandwiches tightly.

Cut them in half, half will be for dinner and half can be for lunch the following day!

I use Frank's hot sauce, this makes it a true buffalo chicken salad!

Hummus Wrap

lavash or pita flat bread
sweet baby romaine
grape tomatoes
peppers
cucumbers
carrots
onions
garbanzo beans
cheddar cheese
hummus

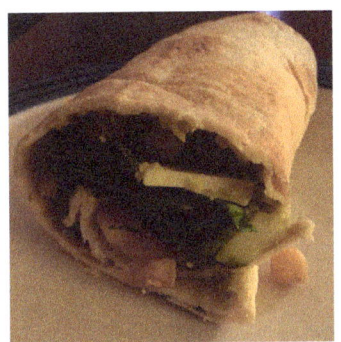

You will notice I didn't give you measurements for this recipe, that's because I want you to buy all the ingredients and try them different ways. Everyone likes them differently, I make them unique for my family. My daughter doesn't like onions, my man doesn't like garbanzo beans, and I tend to make mine as a Hummus Salad for example.

One thing you will do is dice all your ingredients, make them bite-size so this sandwich is easy to eat. I cover the whole bread with my Avocado hummus, Beet Hummus, Garlic Hummus, or my Red Pepper and then add my veggie toppings. This usually becomes a big wrap so I cut it in half, and this is lunch the following day!

Quinoa Cake

2 cups quinoa
2 cups water
2 tsp. paprika
1/2 tsp. cumin
1/2 tsp. oregano
2 eggs, large and beaten
pepper to taste
olive oil to fry

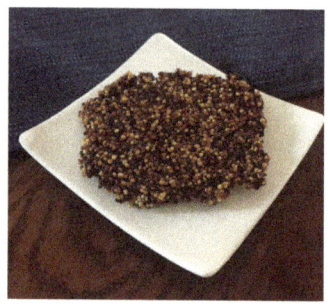

Combine quinoa and water and bring to a boil, reduce heat to low and cover to cook 15–18 minutes or until all water is absorbed. This will cool while you are combining ingredients.

Combine all spices with beaten eggs, now add the cooled quinoa and mix thoroughly. You should have dough that will form into a moist ball. If mix is still dry and fluffy, add a third beaten egg.

Heat pan lightly with olive oil, start with a tablespoon. Form 1/4 cup of mixture into a ball, place in the skillet and flatten with a spatula. Cook for 4 minutes per side till golden brown, add pepper to each cake and serve immediately.

Makes 8 cakes.

Any type of quinoa is fine, here I used tricolor.

Serve over a salad or if you want extra protein, serve with a small piece of wild salmon.

Ranch Chicken Salad Panini

1 loaf rosemary bread
2 chicken breasts
1/2 bottle ranch and chia

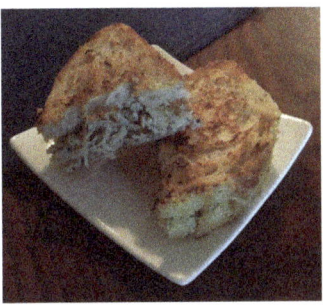

Cook chicken thoroughly, heat olive oil and add raw chicken cubed, or you can boil the chicken and shred it, both ways are good. Make sure the internal temperature is 165 degrees. Once the chicken is thoroughly cooked mix with the ranch and chia dressing over low heat about 10–15 minutes.

Top each sandwich with some chicken, this will make about six sandwiches. I do not heap on the chicken, you should only eat 3 ounces or the size of your palm of any animal protein, so my sandwiches are usually on the thin side but very delicious.

I use a griddle and a pan cover to brown my panini, but if you do not have a griddle you can use a larger pan and a smaller lid to get the same panini effect.

For this recipe we tend to boil the chicken and shred it, please make sure your internal temperature is at least 165 degrees.

Salmon Burger

2 cans wild salmon
1 cup raw organic almonds
6 small green onions, chopped
1 tsp. Italian spices
2 tbsp. lemon juice
2 eggs

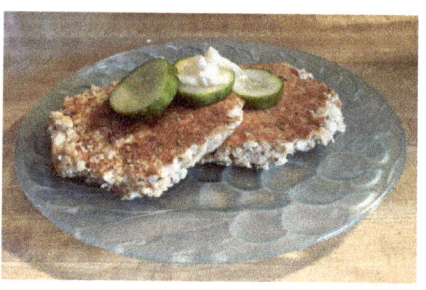

Chop the almonds in a chopper, and mix the salmon in a separate bowl, do not drain the natural juices, mix them into the salmon. Add the almonds to your food processor with the 2 eggs and green onions. Blend for 30 seconds. Now you will add the Italian spices, lemon juice, and salmon. Blend another minute, push ingredients down and blend an extra minute.

Once everything is blended use a spoon to blend by hand, on medium heat add your coconut oil and start spooning out your patties.

I use a teaspoon and make 4 patties at a time. Once you add them to the pan, push them down and form with your spoon the patty.

This recipe makes 10 patties.

I serve them with my homemade pickles!

Tuna Artichoke Melt

2 cans wild albacore tuna
1/2 5 oz. plain Greek yogurt
2 slices onion, chopped
1/2 can artichoke hearts
6 slices Swiss cheese
12 slices rosemary bread

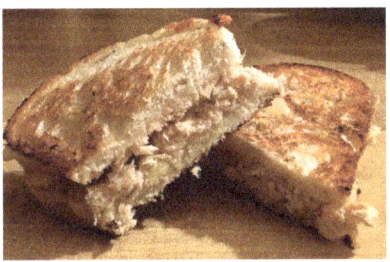

Mix the tuna with the yogurt and the diced onions. I always add the cheese on top of the bread to have the sandwich stick together, but I only use a 1/2 slice on the top and a 1/2 slice on the bottom. My 2nd layer after the cheese will be my artichoke, if you cannot find quartered and only halves, just slice them in to quarters. I line them up usually 6 quarters to cover the sandwich. Now your tuna a scoop on each sandwich, I make 6 sandwiches because these make great lunches the next day.

When purchasing canned artichokes look for artichokes in water. Or you can buy them frozen and cook them yourself.

Tuna Burger

1 tsp. olive oil
1/2 container plain Greek yogurt
2 cans albacore wild tuna
1 tbsp. panko bread crumbs

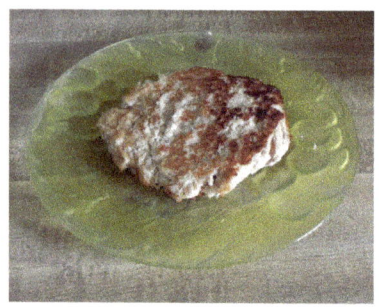

Mix all ingredients together, the tuna I buy is in its natural juices so you do not drain this kind of tuna, you will use the juice too. Heat oil on medium heat for 2 minutes, add 1 heaping tablespoon size of the tuna mixture to the pan. I make 4 burgers at a time and fry them 5 minutes on each side till they have a golden brown look to them.

This recipe will make 4 nice size burgers. I serve them with a side of my garlic kale and a basic salad. I use the single serve organic Greek plain yogurt, and you can add pepper to your mix but you do not need it.

Tuna Salad Sandwich with Pickles

2 cans wild albacore tuna
4 slices Pickles
1/4 brick x-sharp cheddar
6 slices sourdough organic bread

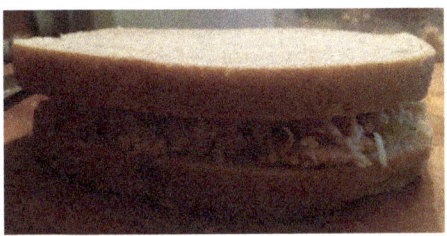

The brand of tuna I buy is in its own natural juices, to utilize the amazing benefits of the omegas in this tuna, you will not drain it, you will mix it all together.

My pickle recipe makes a perfect pairing for this sandwich. I dice these pickles and add them to my tuna before making the sandwich.

I love onions, you can dice some onions or add them individually to the onion lover's sandwiches.

I make this sandwich in two different ways. Just layer it all 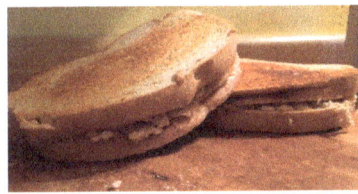 together and serve it cold or make it a panini. I use a square pan, I do not add anything to my pan except the sandwiches 2 or 3 at a time and cover with a lid for about 5 minutes on each side till browned nicely.

Turkey Apple Panini

1 loaf organic rosemary bread
2 organic apples, sliced
1/2 brick organic x-sharp cheddar
1/2 lb. organic turkey

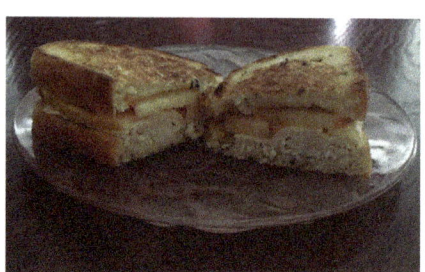

Cut apples in thin slices, I top my bread with 6–7 slices of apples, and then add thinly shredded cheddar to bind the sandwich together. Each sandwich I add 1–2 slices of turkey.

Depending on how much you add to each sandwich this recipe will make between 6–8 sandwiches. And make great leftover lunches.

I do not add anything to my pan, I heat 3 sandwiches at a time and cover them with a smaller lid then my pan to create a panini type sandwich. Each sandwich will need about 5 minutes on each side to get a golden brown look and not burn on medium high heat.

I like to use the organic rosemary bread but organic sourdough bread works great too! I also like using either oven roasted or smoked organic turkey slices.

To get the best flavor out of this sandwich, make sure to use an extra sharp cheddar.

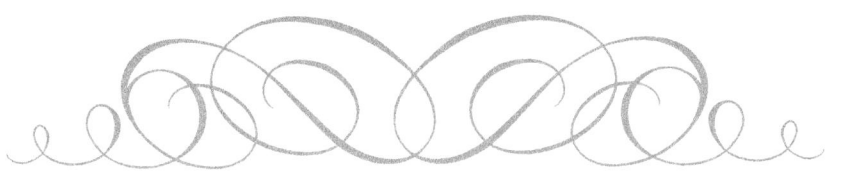

Meals

Thank you *God* for the world so *Sweet*,
Thank you for the *Food* we eat,
Thank you for the *Birds* that sing,
Thank you God for *Everything!*
Amen.

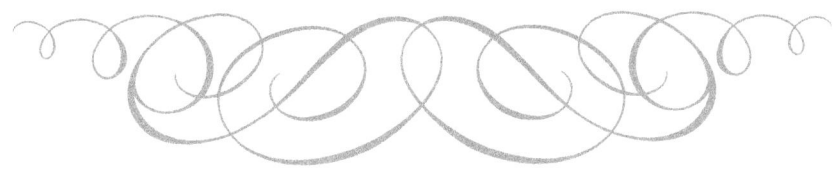

I do not believe in dieting but I have always tended to eat similar to intermittent fasting even before I knew what intermittent fasting was. Not as strict as most as you can see, mostly making sure my body has enough time to thoroughly digest every meal.

Upon waking I drink my ACV Water, I get my family and myself ready for the day and three hours later I usually drink my Healthy Fat Shake. I do not eat anything until lunch, I only drink water. Lunch is usually around noontime and is usually a salad with a healthy fat like avocado and a protein like beans, if I have carbs I usually have them for lunch. I always give my body time to digest and utilize what I eat. I don't drink with my meals and will drink water a half an hour before and after my meals. If I come home hungry, which does happen from time to time, I tend to eat nuts or a spoonful of almond butter, this helps me stay away from snacking while preparing dinner. My dinners are usually around 6:00 p.m., and that is when I serve proteins with vegetables. Dinner is my last meal of the night. My body needs time to do what it needs to do before I go to sleep.

You may think this is pretty strict, but for me it is not, it has been a work in progress for years to get to this point. And through the things I have gone through I try very hard to treat my body the best way I can so it can repair itself more easily as I age. Am I perfect? No, but I try my best! Do I have days where I fall away from my routine? Yes, I do, but I don't let it derail me, I get back on track the next day and try not to dwell on it.

Okay, now on to the main dishes. These may take a bit longer to prepare but trust me they will be worth the time, effort, and love you will put into making them!

Broccoli Quinoa Bake

1 1/2 cups quinoa
3 cups water
1 pkg. broccoli, frozen
1 8 oz. extra sharp cheddar
1/2 small garlic clove, minced
pepper to taste

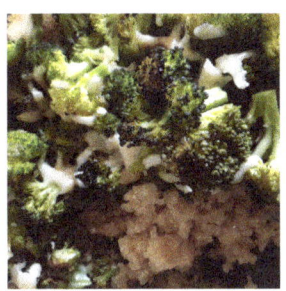

Mince garlic and add it to a glass baking dish that you have pregreased with coconut oil. Mix in the frozen broccoli, if you do not like big florets you can chop them prior.

Cook quinoa according to package directions, once cooked transfer it to the glass baking dish. Grate cheddar and mix in 1/2 of it, bake at 350 for 15 minutes. Mix well and top with the remaining cheddar. Bake for an additional 5–10 minutes until cheese is melted.

I add pepper, about a tsp. should do!

Cauliflower Alfredo

1 head cauliflower, chopped
7–8 cloves garlic, chopped
1/2 cup water
1/2 cup parmesan, grated
pepper to taste

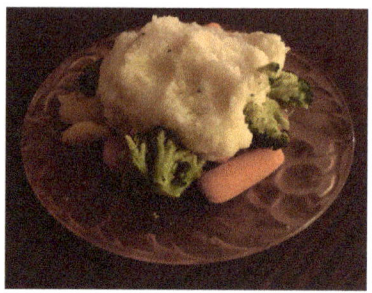

Cut cauliflower in florets, place in a pot with the water and garlic, cook until tender about 10–15 minutes. Let cool before blending, I puree the cauliflower, garlic and leftover water with the Parmesan (I use Pecorino Romano in mine). You may have to add a little more water, blend and see how the texture is and add water a little at a time.

Use right away or pour into jars and use later in the week.

This is great over veggies like pictured, or vegetable noodles, or even tortellini!

Cauliflower Fried Rice

1 head cauliflower
1/2 cup peas, frozen
1 onion, diced
1/4 cup corn
1/4 cup carrots, diced
1 tbsp. olive oil
6 eggs
1/4 cup almond milk
1/2 tsp. lemon pepper

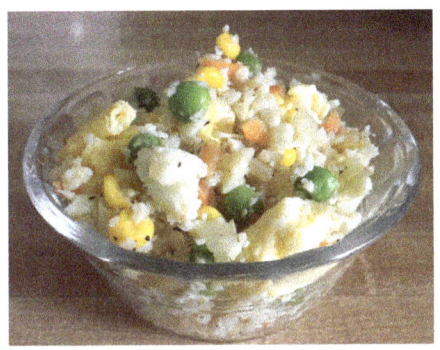

Wash and cut cauliflower into florets, place in a food processor, and pulse a few times until you reach rice consistency.

Heat oil in a large skillet and add diced onion, stirring often until translucent but not browned. Add cauliflower "rice," frozen peas, diced carrots, and corn kernels. Stirring often about 10-15 minutes until heated through.

Reduce heat to low and prepare your scrambled eggs. Whisk the 6 eggs with the ¼ cup almond milk till combined well.

Pour the scrambled eggs in a coconut-oiled pan and chop into smaller pieces to be added to your fried "rice." Once egg is prepared, add lemon pepper to your cauliflower "rice" and stir on medium heat.

I add the egg per plate, but if everyone likes eggs you can add it in your skillet and stir before serving.

Cauliflower Pizza Crust

1/2 head cauliflower (2 cups)
1 clove garlic, minced
1 cup fresh mozzarella
1 egg, beaten
1 tsp. basil
1 tsp. oregano

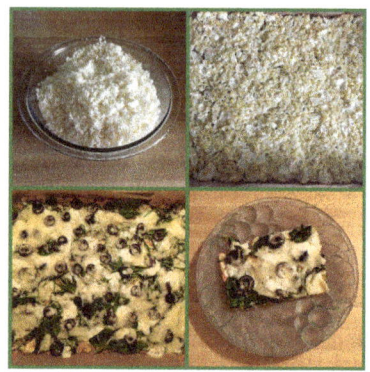

Preheat oven to 400 degrees, prep a cookie sheet or pizza stone, make sure to grease it so it doesn't stick. Or you can use parchment paper but it may not crust the same.

Prep your cauliflower—wash and remove stems and leaves, and cut into florets. Add to a food processor and pulse until the texture is similar to rice. If you do not have a food processor, you can use a box cheese grater. Sauté cauliflower "rice" over medium heat, cook until translucent approximately 6–8 minutes. In a bowl combine the cauliflower rice with the remaining ingredients.

Spread dough evenly, about 1/4"–1/3" thick and the pizza should be about 9"–10" in diameter. Bake 25–30 minutes or until the crust is golden. Remove the crust from the oven and top with pizza sauce and your toppings but do not add too many heavy toppings, as you do not want to weigh down the pizza. Broil for 5 more minutes or until the toppings are hot and cheese is melted. Allow the pizza to cool 2–3 minutes before cutting and serve immediately. Pictured I used spinach, olives, and mozzarella cheese on this pizza.

Chicken Asparagus Bake

4 tbsp. butter
4 tbsp. garbanzo bean flour
1 1/2 cups chicken broth
8 oz. mushrooms, sliced
2 lg. chicken breasts, cooked
1 lb. asparagus
1/4 cup panko
2 tbsp. almonds, chopped
extra melted butter

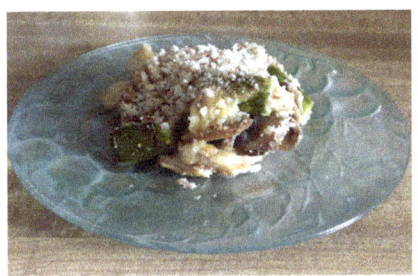

Slice and cook your chicken with extra virgin olive oil, make sure the internal temperature is 165 degrees, cook through. Make a rue with the butter and flour, add chicken broth and stir until thickened. In a separate bowl add your panko, chopped almonds, and melted butter. Stir till combined. In a glass baking dish coat with coconut oil, now add the cooked chicken, 1/2 the sauce and the cooked asparagus in layers. Add the mushrooms and the remaining sauce. Top with the panko mixture.

Bake 20 minutes on 375 degrees.

I do not like mushrooms so I add them to only 1/2 of my pan. You can add 1 tsp. of black pepper to the sauce if you would like.

Chicken Cacciatore

2 squash, chopped
1/2 bag baby carrots, chopped
1/2 onion, chopped
3 tomatoes, diced
1 tbsp. Italian spices
1 can crushed tomatoes
4 chicken breasts, skinless and boneless

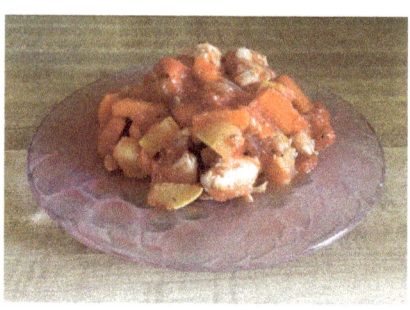

Prepare your chicken in small cubes. Cook the chicken in a large skillet with olive oil, make sure the internal temperature is 165 degrees. In a large pot add all of the vegetables and the can of crushed tomatoes. Sprinkle with the Italian spices and cook on medium heat about 20 minutes, in the meantime your chicken will be cooking and once the chicken is cooked entirely through you can add it to the pot of vegetables.

This recipe is made to be chunky, add more vegetables if need be. And plan on this having leftovers.

This recipe I use these vegetables but sometimes add peppers and/or zucchini. It depends on what vegetables I have available.

Chicken Souvlaki

2 lg. chicken breasts, cooked
3 cups sweet baby romaine
1/2 tomato, diced
1/4 onion, diced
1 red, yellow, and orange peppers
1 tbsp. Greek dressing, each salad
12 black olives, sliced
feta cheese

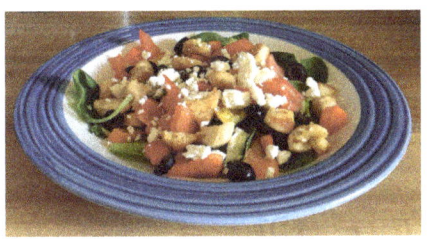

Slice and cook your chicken with extra virgin olive oil, make sure the internal temperature is 165 degrees, cook through. While the chicken is cooking dice all the vegetables and prepare your plates with the lettuce. I add the chicken last and then top it with my Greek dressing.

I use red, yellow, and orange bell peppers but you can use any kind you like. A true souvlaki uses green peppers. I also use black olives but a true souvlaki uses kalamta olives.

Spinach Artichoke Falafel

3–4 cups (5 oz.) spinach
2 shallots
3 cloves garlic
1 14 oz. artichoke hearts
2 15 oz. garbanzo beans
1 tbsp. lemon juice
2 1/2 tsp. ground cumin
2 tsp. ground coriander
1/2 tsp. paprika
1/4 tsp. oregano dried
1/8 tsp. cayenne pepper
1 pinch ground black pepper
1/4 cup garbanzo bean flour

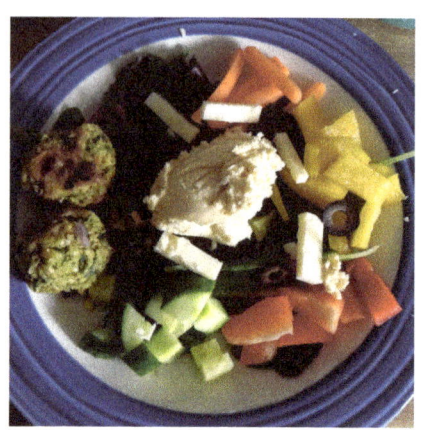

Preheat the oven to 350 degrees. Line two baking sheets with parchment paper.

In a blender or food processor combine the spinach, chopped shallots, and chopped garlic. Add the drained artichoke hearts, lemon juice, and spices, and blend to incorporate. Add the chickpea and chickpea flour, pulse until the chickpeas reach a very crumbly but not smooth texture. If the mixture is too thin to form into balls, stir in more chickpea flour, but do not blend any longer.

Scooping a tablespoon at a time form a ball on your parchment paper, and flatten slightly. Repeat until all the mixture is used 12 on each baking sheet. Bake for 20–25 minutes or until firm enough to flip. Bake another 20 minutes on the other side, until browned and slightly crisp on the outside. Let cool a few minutes before removing from pan to avoid breaking.

Farro

1 cup farro
3 cups water
1 28 oz. can fire roasted crushed tomatoes
2 15 oz. cans garbanzo beans
1/4 cup Pecorino Romano cheese, grated

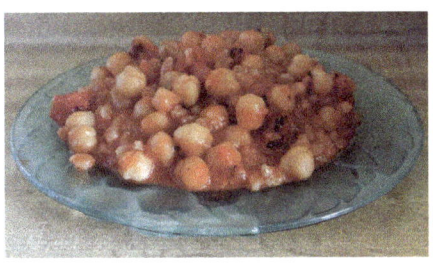

Cook farro as directed. Add tomatoes and drained garbanzo beans and continue to simmer with 1/4 cup cheese. Simmer about 5–10 minutes until heated through.

Serve with a salad and a little extra cheese on top.

A simple dish my family loves, and if you have someone who does not like garbanzo beans (chick peas) they will love them in this recipe!

Lazy Lasagna Bake

1 clove garlic, minced
2 zucchini, diced
1/4 cup onion, diced
1 pkg. rice pasta spirals
1/2 batch Momma's Sauce
1/4 batch Momma's Ricotta
1/2 cup fresh mozzarella, diced
1/4 cup Pecorino Romano, grated

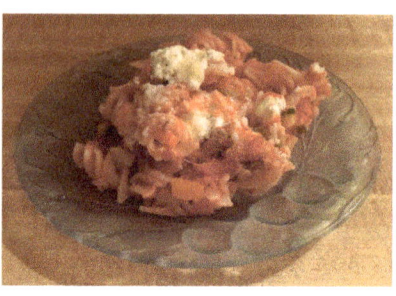

Sauté zucchini and onion with garlic, you do not need to add oil because the zucchini is a wet vegetable, let the mixture sweat and constantly stir so it does not burn about 15 minutes or until translucent on medium heat.

Add Momma's sauce and continue cooking for 10 minutes while you are cooking the pasta. Follow the pasta cooking instructions, I bring the water to a rapid boil before adding the pasta and cook it for 15 minutes until al dente.

Drain the pasta and mix the pasta with the sauce. Now add a layer of plain sauce to your stockpot, then a layer of the pasta zucchini mix and droplets of ricotta and mozzarella. Continue layering until all ingredients are used. Cover your pot and simmer for 10 minutes until cheese is melted.

You can use summer squash and eggplant in this recipe, too, if they are in season you know I am using them!

Lazy Pierogi

1 pkg. rice spiral pasta
1 cream of mushroom soup
1/2–3/4 cup sauerkraut
1/4–1/2 tsp. pepper

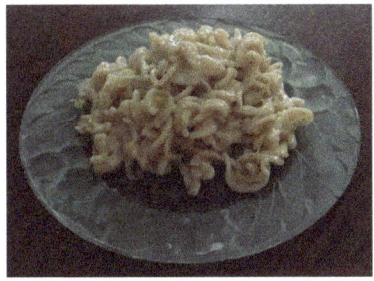

Make pasta according to directions, once cooked to al dente you will drain and keep aside. In the same pot heat the cream of mushroom soup and then add the pasta and sauerkraut and mix well.

Serve immediately.

I like sauerkraut but not everyone does so start with a 1/2 cup and add more if you desire.

I use rice pasta for this recipe.

This is lazy cooking so I do use boxed organic gluten free cream of mushroom soup.

Loaded Sweet Potato

3 lbs. sweet potatoes
kale
1 can black beans, drained
Guacamole

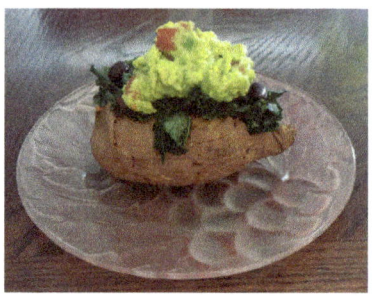

Preheat your oven to 400 degrees, I bake a 3-lb. bag of sweet potatoes, this will be about 9 medium-sized potatoes. Pierce each potato with a fork 3 times on each side and bake for 45–50 minutes.

Meanwhile, make your garlic kale. Also make your guacamole.

Once your potatoes are baked and your toppings are prepared you will layer them like the picture.

This dish will become one of your favorites and you will prepare extra for lunch the next day!

Pierogi

3 cups organic all-purpose flour
3/4 cup boiling water
1/4 cup cold water
1 tsp. olive oil

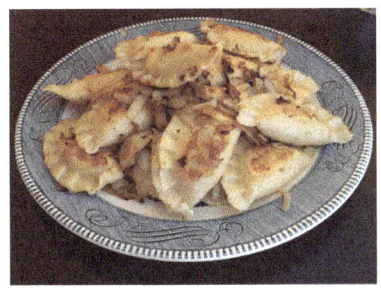

Mix 3 cups flour and 3/4 cup boiling water either by hand or on a food processor. Cover with cotton cloth or lid from food processor for 5 minutes.

Add 1/4 cup cold water, mix, cover, and let stand 15 minutes.

Add 1 tsp. olive oil and blend, if not dough yet add less than 1/4 cup of water till it is pliable.

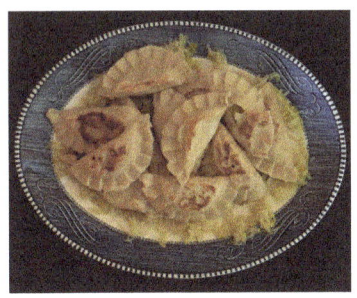

Now knead and roll, I cut dough in fourths and roll out, cut circles with either a cookie cutter or a lid, collect scraps, knead and roll again.

I use a crimper to make it easier, fill with sauerkraut, farmer's cheese or a potato cheddar mixture.

This recipe will make about 24.

Once the pierogis are all made, boil a pot of water when it reaches a rolling boil add six pierogi at a time to cook. They will get bigger and start to float, stir consistently for about 5-6 minutes. Once cooled you can freeze them for later use. When you are ready to use them, if frozen boil again and melt 1-tablespoon butter with cooked onions in a frying pan add 5 pierogis at a time to brown on each side.

Salsa Quinoa Bake

1 cup quinoa
2 cups water
Momma's salsa
Frank's (optional)

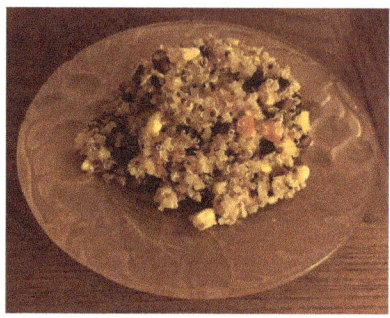

Cook quinoa according to package. Once cooked add my salsa to it and mix thoroughly.

Serves 4-6.

You can use regular or tri-colored quinoa, both work wonderfully. This will not be spicy, so we add Frank's.

Spinach and Squash Mini Manicotti

4 oz. spinach, frozen
1 whole roasted acorn squash
8 oz. ricotta cheese
manicotti Shells, small
Momma's Sauce

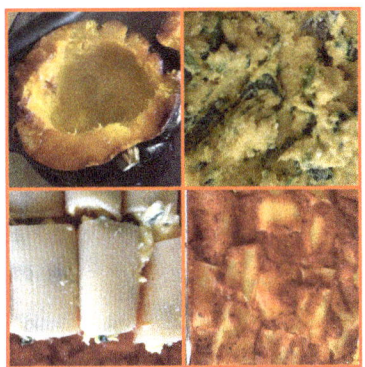

    Mix ingredients together while you are precooking the shells till they are al dente so you can handle them and not crack them while stuffing. Add roasted acorn squash to your ricotta mix, the spinach will defrost in the mix.

    Once shells are warm not hot and you can touch them start stuffing them with a small spoon. Place on a bed of your sauce, I use a glass baking pan.

    Top the manicotti with more sauce and bake at 400 degrees for 20 minutes or until pasta is cooked through.

    I use small manicotti shells but you can use any size shells. My recipe made 24 small manicottis.

Squash Mac and Cheese

1–1 1/2 lbs. butternut squash
1 12 oz. pkg. kale or spinach, frozen
1 1/2 cups almond milk
1 1/2 cups x-sharp cheddar
1/4 cup Pecorino Romano
1 pkg. spiral rice pasta, cooked
1/4 cup panko bread crumbs

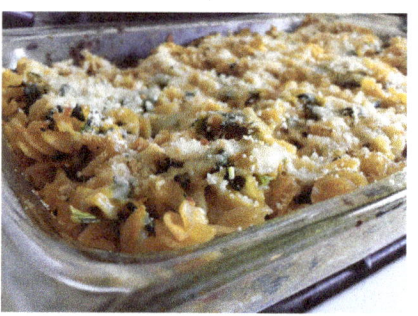

You can roast a whole squash prior to this meal or cut it in chunks and simmer it on the stove top with the almond milk for 12 minutes until softened. Be careful to the heat so it won't boil over, keep 1/2 covered while simmering. While cooking your squash, boil the water for your pasta and cook according to its directions, you will want your pasta al dente because you will be baking it also. Once butternut squash is cooked, mash it with the remaining almond milk, now add the shredded cheddar and continue to mash, you will see it get creamier now.

Prep a glass baking dish with coconut oil, in the pot you boiled the pasta add the drained pasta and mix in some of the squash mix. I do this in stages adding pasta, frozen kale, grated Romano, squash, and continue mixing.

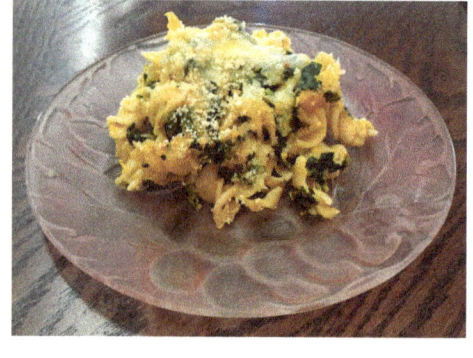

Now that everything is combined, if you feel you need it a little creamier you can add 1/4 cup more almond milk, if not top with remaining cheddar and panko. Bake 15 minutes or until cheese is melted.

Vegetable Lasagna

2 zucchini, medium
2 yellow squash, medium
3 carrots, medium
2 cups broccoli, fresh
Momma's Sauce
Momma's Ricotta
1 cup mozzarella, shredded

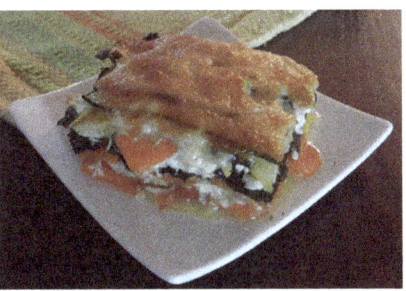

If you have a mandolin, slice all your vegetables lengthwise and cut your broccoli in very small pieces.

Prepare your glass baking dish with coconut oil and preheat the oven to 350 degrees.

Add Momma's sauce to the bottom of the pan and now start layering one vegetable at a time. Once you have layered all the vegetables add droplets of the ricotta mixture being sure to spread it along the whole lasagna.

You will continue to layer like this starting with the sauce, then the vegetables, and finally the ricotta until everything is used and you reach the top of your baking dish. I usually make 3 layers.

Top your lasagna with mozzarella and bake for 30 minutes. It will have water from the vegetables in the bottom, you can drain it prior to serving.

Pictured I did not use my sauce and it came out amazing too!

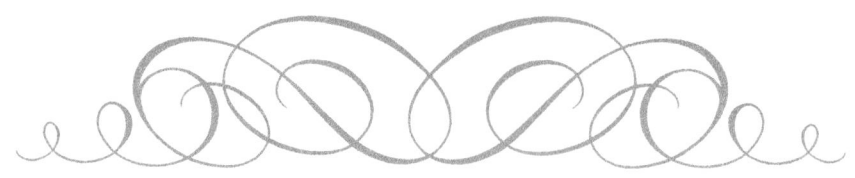

Condiments

Taste and *See* how good the *Lord* is;
happy the man who takes refuge in him.

—Psalms 34:9

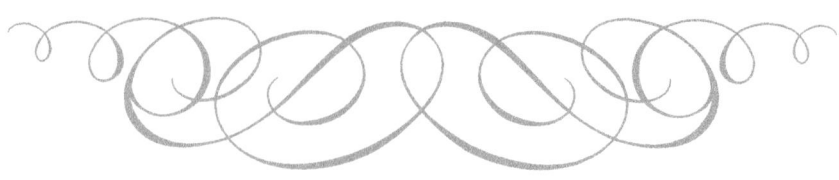

LIVE NATURALLY

Now with some of my recipes you have noticed you may need some ingredients I did not include. That's because I make them from scratch. I started doing this many years ago because the products that I used to buy started constantly changing ingredients. And some products I would notice the ingredient lists changing almost monthly, to me that is disturbing. I tend to trust products that I buy, but when I see them adding foreign ingredients so they can keep it on the shelf longer, I stop buying them.

I would notice the many different words they would use to add sugar, have you ever noticed how many there are? Let me list them in alphabetical order for you since this list is lengthy!

Agave nectar, aspartame, Barbados sugar, barley malt, barley malt syrup, beet sugar, brown sugar, buttered sugar, cane juice, cane juice crystals, cane sugar, caramel, carob syrup, castor sugar, coconut palm sugar, coconut sugar, confectioners sugar, corn sweetener, corn syrup, corn syrup solids, date sugar, dehydrated cane juice, demerara sugar, dextrin, dextrose, diatase, diastatic malt, ethyl maltol, evaporated cane juice, free flowing brown sugars, fructose, fruit juice, fruit juice concentrate, Florida crystals, glactose, glucose, glucose solid, golden sugar, golden syrup, grape sugar, high fructose corn syrup (HFCS), honey, icing sugar, invert sugar, lactose, maltodextrin, maltol, maltose, malt sugar, mannitol, mannose, maple syrup, molasses, muscovado, palm sugar, panocha, powdered sugar, raw sugar, refiner's syrup, rice sugar, rice syrup, saccharose, sorbitol, sorghum, sucrose, sugar (granulated), sweet sorghum, syrup, treacle, turbinado sugar, and yellow sugar.

And this list is ever growing!

And sugar isn't the only thing they add to products to keep their shelf life stable.

You will notice with my condiments, sugar is never added! And, yes, you will need to use these within a week or two, but you will be happy knowing it is fresh all of the time. And trust me, they probably won't even last that long, you will be making them more often like I do. The taste of my condiments you can't find in the stores. They have become staples in my household and I hope they become staples in yours!

Avocado Hummus

1 15.5 oz. can garbanzo beans
1/4 cup lemon juice
1 tbsp. olive oil
2 cloves garlic, chopped
2 ripe avocados cut in chunks
1 dash cumin
2 tbsp. cilantro

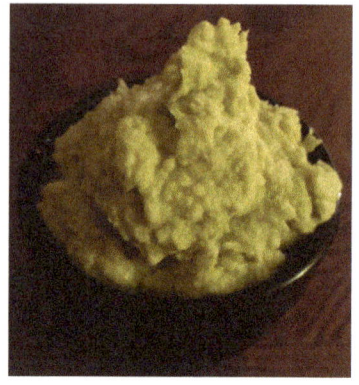

In a food processor add drained garbanzo beans with the rest of the ingredients and blend. If hummus is too thick add a tsp. of water. Blend until smooth, you may need to stop and push sides down to mix completely.

That's it! Enjoy!

Serve with vegetables.

Beet Hummus

1 small roasted beet
1 15.5 oz. can garbanzo beans
zest of a lemon
juice of half a large lemon
pinch of pepper
2 cloves garlic, large and minced
1/4 cup olive oil

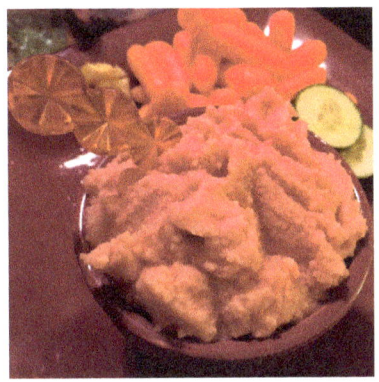

Once your beet is cooled and peeled, quarter it and place it in your food processor. Blend until only small bits remain. Add remaining ingredients except for olive oil and blend until smooth. Drizzle in the olive oil as the hummus is mixing, taste and adjust seasonings as needed. If it is too thick, add a little water and continue to blend until smooth.

Will keep in the fridge for up to a week.

See beet roasting instructions on Roasted Beets.

Garlic Hummus

1 can 15.5 oz. garbanzo beans
1/4 cup lemon juice
1 tbsp. olive oil
2 cloves garlic

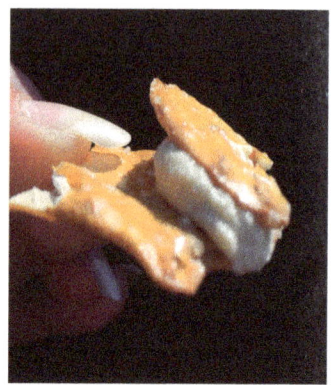

Drain beans and add all ingredients in a food processor and blend until smooth, you may have to push down the sides and blend again so everything mixes properly.

Depending on how much you and your guests love garlic will depend on the size cloves you use, 2 large ones will make this recipe very garlicky, so if you do not like strong garlic, start with either 2 small cloves or 1 large clove. You can taste it and decide if you would like to add more.

Greek Dressing

1 clove garlic, large and minced
1 tsp. Italian seasonings
1/4 tsp. ground pepper
1/4 cup lemon juice
1/2 cup olive oil

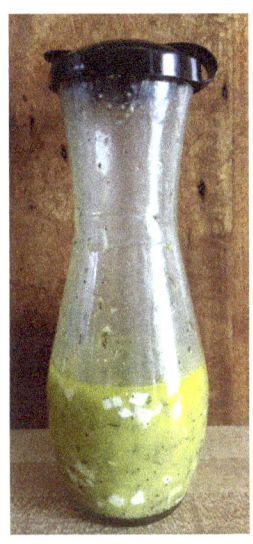

    Add all ingredients in a glass dressing bottle or a glass mason jar. Put lid on and shake vigorously. Store in the fridge and when you are ready to use it take it out 10–15 minutes prior to warm up solidified oil. If you need it faster, you can run it under warm to hot water a few minutes and shake till liquefied.

    I prefer freshly squeezed lemon juice but if lemons are not in season you can use bottled pure lemon juice.

    If you do not have Italian seasoning blend, oregano works well in this recipe also.

Guacamole

2 ripe Avocado
¼ cup Red Onion, chopped
½ Lemon, squeezed
½ Tomato, chopped
2 Cloves Garlic, minced

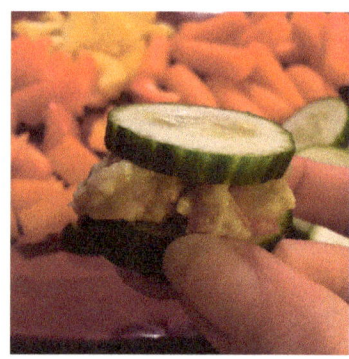

Chop all vegetables and add to a food processor, mix in lemon juice. You can hand mash this, I have but my food processor makes it a bit creamier.

Serve with vegetables or chips.

Momma's Sauce

2 28 oz. cans fire roasted crushed tomatoes
14 baby carrots, finely chopped
1 red pepper, finely chopped
1/2 zucchini, finely chopped
1/2 yellow squash, finely chopped
1/4 red onion, finely chopped
2–3 cloves garlic, small and minced
Italian spices

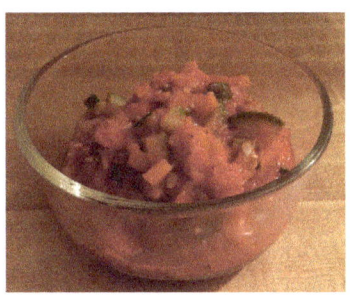

Chop all vegetables and add to the tomatoes in a large pot. Add spices, I do not measure it is all by eye, make sure spices are all over the top of the mixture. Mix together now and add more spices the same way and mix again.

Simmer an hour to an hour and a half.

Water from veggies will rise to the top, mix it together the first few times. Some vegetables different times of the year may hold more water than others, if you have a lot of water after doing this a few times you can spoon some out.

Pesto

4 cups spinach, raw about 3 oz.
1 clove garlic, large and chopped
1/2 cup olive oil
1/4 cup almonds, raw and chopped
1/4 cup Pecorino Romano, grated

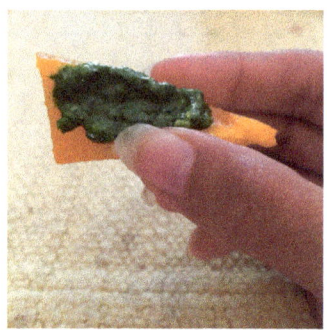

In a chopper, chop almonds and add them to the food processor with the spinach, garlic, olive oil, and Romano cheese. Blend until completely combined, you may need to stop it and scrape the sides down and blend a second time till smooth.

Pickles

6 mini cucumbers
6–8 cloves garlic
1 onion, sliced
2 cups apple cider vinegar
2 cup water

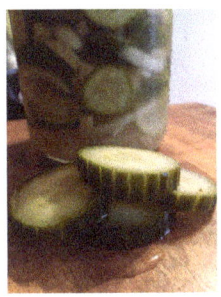

Wash and dry your cucumbers, cut the top and bottom off and cut in thick slices. Slice a whole onion and dice your garlic cloves.

Make the brine, combine the water and apple cider vinegar and bring to a boil.

Layer your mason jar with onion, garlic, and cucumbers making sure they are tightly packed. Cool the brine a bit and then fill your jar leaving 1/4 of an inch at the top. Place the lid on the jar but do not screw it on, the mixture needs to breath. Wait 10–15 minutes and then tighten the lid and refrigerate. I keep them refrigerated 3 weeks before eating, and they will keep a few months but they probably won't last. The onions and garlic taste amazing in this recipe too!!

Any size of cucumbers work, and you can slice them in spears also just make sure you completely pack the jar before adding the brine. I don't add sea salt but if you do use 1 tsp.

Red Pepper Hummus

2 cans garbanzo beans
1 12 oz. jar roasted red peppers
1/4 cup olive oil

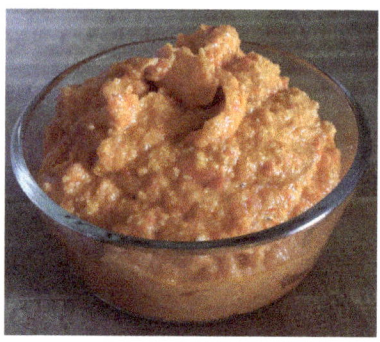

    Chop roasted red peppers and add all ingredients to a food processor and blend thoroughly. If it is not smooth add a tablespoon more olive oil, push ingredients down in blender and continue to blend.

    You will only need to blend 5 minutes at most, listen to the blender it will tell you when you need to stop and push the ingredients down.

    I usually blend twice just to make sure it is as smooth as I like it.

Ricotta Cheese Mixture

16 oz. container Ricotta cheese
3/4 cup Pecorino Romano cheese
8 slices provolone, diced (1cup)
1 tbsp. Italian seasonings

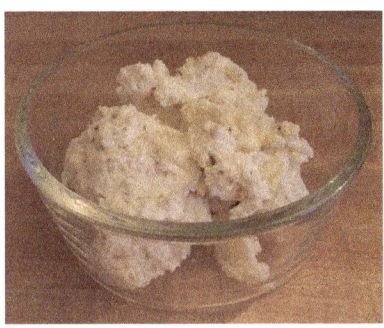

    Dice provolone and add it to the rest of the cheeses and spices. Mix well to combine.

    I use whole milk ricotta, but have used part skim and they come out the same. I have also used garlic and herb spices if I don't have Italian spices and it works well too.

    This mixture will make a whole lasagna, will fill manicotti or stuffed shells, but I also use it on my Rosabella Pizza and 1/2 of this mixture in my Lazy Lasagna recipe.

Salsa

1 cup tomatoes, chopped
1/2 cup red pepper, diced
1/4 cup onion, diced
1/2 cup black beans, drained
1/2 cup corn, husked
1/4 tsp. cumin
1/4 tsp. cayenne
1/4 tsp. cilantro

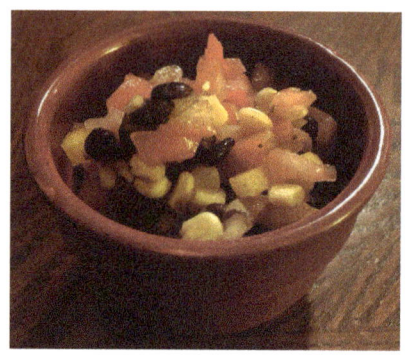

Chop and dice all vegetables and add to a bowl, drain black beans and add to the vegetables. Add spices and mix well.

Refrigerate or serve immediately.

I have used tomatoes on the vine but if grape tomatoes are only available, they work nicely too!

I only use organic corn from my organic farm share. I husk and cook it when I receive it in the summer and freeze most of it for the winter.

Vinaigrette

3 tbsps. olive oil
2 tbsps. apple cider vinegar
1/2 tsps. garlic and herb spices

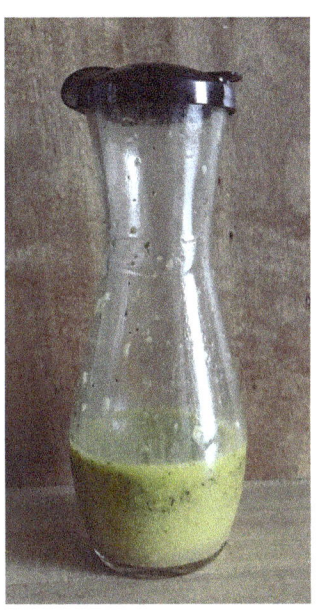

Add all ingredients to a bottle like this or a mason jar, put the lid on and shake vigorously.

This will serve 6 salads.

Pour this whole recipe on chopped cucumbers, tomatoes, peppers, onions, and celery. Refrigerate for 20 minutes before serving either by itself or on a bed of romaine.

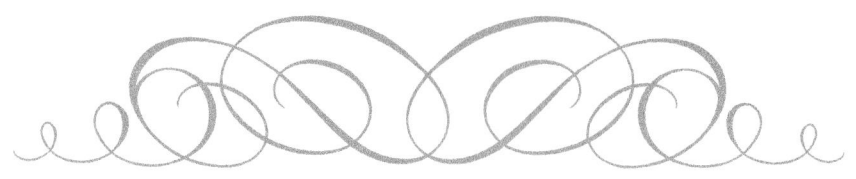

Party Time

Be truly glad—there is wonderful *Joy* ahead!

—1 Peter 1:6

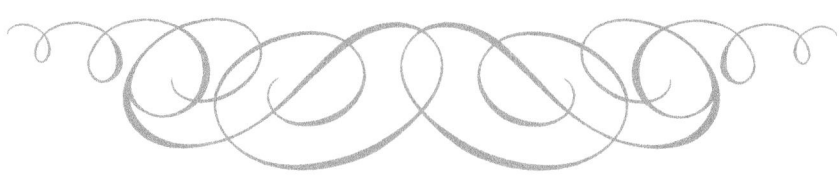

In case you didn't know, I really enjoy cooking and feeding my family and friends the best food available to me. My family entertains once a week sometimes more in the summer time. The staples I always include are any two items in my condiments section of this book. And a few items in this section as well. But the main dishes I serve them as I am preparing everything else, can you guess?

Yes, you are right! A fruit tray especially in the summertime and always a veggie tray! I have these out right away before I serve anything else, do they know the reason why, no, probably not, but if you have read this book up until now I am sure you know the reason I do!

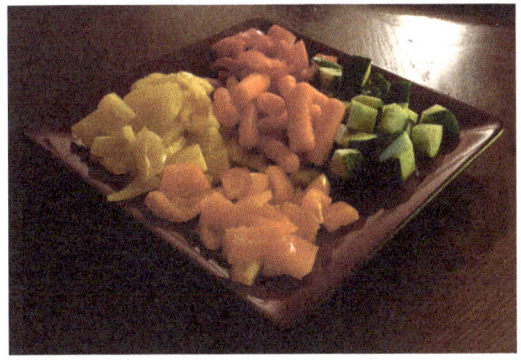

So, before you even say it, I already know what your reaction to this section will be!

You are probably like wait, what? All this talk about wheat and protein not mixing with starches and you feed your family and friends homemade pizza? Well, I cannot change anyone and we are from an area outside of Buffalo, NY, and New Yorkers are known for their pizza. So, yes, I make pizza and if you ask anyone of my family and friends they will say mine is the best! You will notice a few different things from my pizzas versus the typical pizza.

I chose the best dough, yes, only 3 ingredients at my local bakery that is made fresh daily and I top it with quality ingredients some of which my guests would probably never purchase let alone eat. But at my house they open their mind to new foods and have never complained!

Buffalo Wing Dip

1 8 oz. cream cheese
1/4 cup blue cheese crumbles
1/2 cup plain Greek yogurt
juice from 1/2 of a lemon
1 tbsp. apple cider vinegar
1/4 tsp. garlic powder
1/4 tsp. onion powder
1/4 tsp. black pepper
1/2 cup hot sauce
1/2 cup mozzarella
2 cups cooked chicken, diced
1/4 –1/2 cup mozzarella

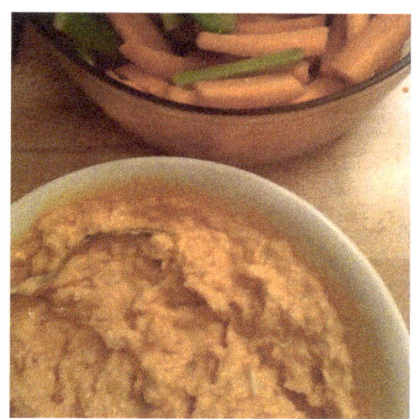

Preheat oven to 300 degrees. Combine blue cheese crumbles, plain Greek yogurt, lemon juice, ACV, garlic powder, onion powder, and black pepper. This will become your healthier version of blue cheese dressing.

In a separate bowl combine cream cheese and hot sauce, the cream cheese will still be clumpy. Add your blue cheese mixture, chicken and 1/2 cup mozzarella. Mix till everything is combined.

Use an 8x8" glass pie pan and bake for 20 minutes, pull out and give it a good mix and now add the extra 1/2 cup of mozzarella to the top. Continue to bake till cheese is melted and starting to brown.

I only use Frank's hot sauce. I recently changed this recipe to chopped celery and carrots instead of the chicken; it is up to you!

Serve with carrots and celery or avocado oil potato chips.

Buffalo Wing Pizza

1 bakery pizza dough
1/2 cup carrots, diced
1/2 cup celery, diced
1/4 cup blue cheese crumbles
1 1/2 cups chicken, cooked
2 cups mozzarella

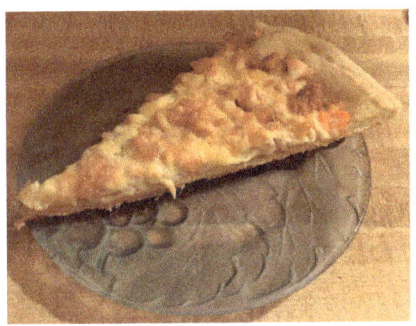

Preheat your pizza stone in an oven of 400 degrees for 20 minutes, I do this while I am prepping my pizzas.

Dice the vegetables fine, they will have a crunch so I make mine small and spread it to cover the whole pizza, do the same with the celery and the chicken. The blue cheese I don't add a lot but you taste it in every bite. Top with mozzarella.

Cook your pizza for 20 minutes or until cheese is melted and crust is browned.

Add some Frank's to your slice always makes it taste best!

Pesto Pizza

1 bakery pizza dough
Momma's pesto
5 oz. fresh mozzarella, cubed
12 grape tomatoes, sliced
1/4 cup Romano cheese, grated

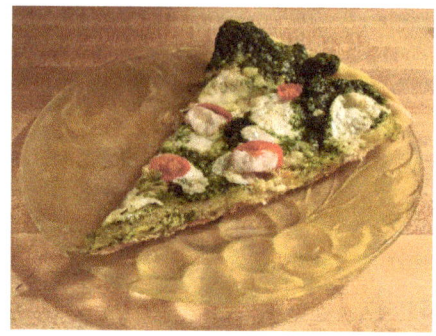

Preheat your pizza stone in an oven of 400 degrees for 20 minutes, I do this while I am prepping my pizzas.

I use 1/2 my pesto recipe to cover this pizza and top it with sliced tomatoes, cubed fresh mozzarella and shake the grated Romano over the whole pizza.

Cook your pizza for 20 minutes or until cheese is melted and crust is browned.

You can slice roma tomatoes or on the vine, tomatoes taste amazing with this recipe also.

Rosabella Pizza

1 bakery pizza dough
1 clove garlic, minced
2 cups spinach, raw
16 grape tomatoes, sliced
1/2 cup ricotta mixture
1/4 cup onions, sliced (optional)
2 cups mozzarella, shredded
olive oil

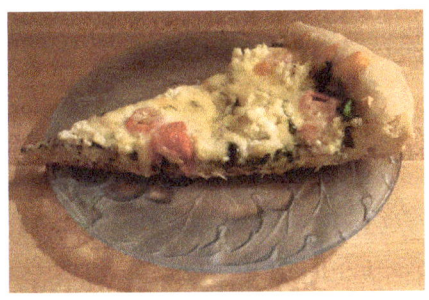

Preheat your pizza stone in an oven of 400 degrees for 20 minutes, I do this while I am prepping my pizzas.

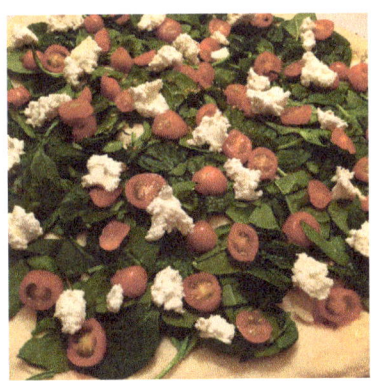

Once pizza dough is spread on stone drizzle olive oil all over pizza dough. Spread garlic over pizza, little pieces everywhere. Rough chop the raw spinach and spread over pizza, it will look like a lot but it cooks down. Add sliced grape tomatoes and little droplets of the ricotta mixture. Now top with your mozzarella and onions.

Cook your pizza for 20 minutes or until cheese is melted and crust is browned.

I add onions to the top 1/2 of the pizza as not everyone likes onions, but they taste delicious with this pizza.

Spinach Artichoke Avocado Dip

12 oz. spinach, frozen
1 1/2 cups artichokes, frozen
4 oz. cream cheese
1 ripe avocado
4 cloves garlic, minced
1 tbsp. olive oil
1/2 cup Parmesan, grated
1/4 cup Gruyere, shredded

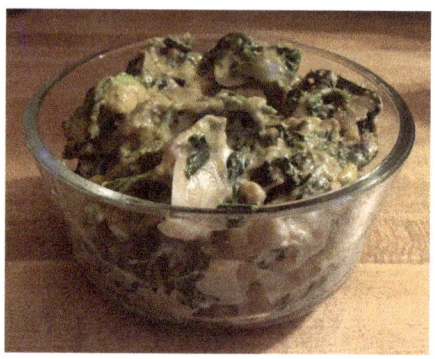

Preheat the oven to 375 degrees. Sauté minced garlic and olive oil for about 1 minute, making sure garlic does not burn. Add the spinach and artichokes and continue to sauté for 5 minutes.

You can chop the artichokes prior to this or once the mixture is cooked.

In a bowl combine the cream cheese and avocado, mash until smooth and mixed completely. Stir in 1/4 cup Parmesan and the Gruyere. Transfer to a coconut or olive oil greased glass baking dish. Top with the rest of the Parmesan cheese. Bake for 15 minutes.

I have used kale in this recipe and it tasted amazing, you can also use Swiss chard, or collard greens!

Spinach Artichoke Dip

Alfredo Recipe

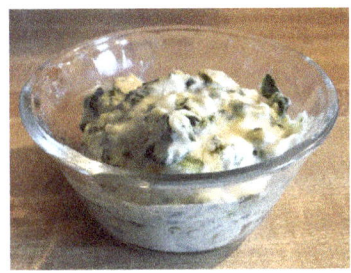

1 tbsp. butter
1 tbsp. garbanzo bean flour
2 cups almond milk
1/2 cup Pecorino Romano, grated

Dip Mix

4–6 cloves roasted garlic
1 10 oz. pkg. frozen spinach
1 14 oz. can artichoke hearts
1/3 cup Pecorino Romano, grated
1 cup Mozzarella, diced
1 pkg. Neufchatel organic cream cheese

Roast garlic for 20 minutes at 350 degrees, just trim top and bottom before roasting. The skins will slip off easily and then you will mince.

Make rue with the butter and flour, slowly add milk over low heat. Once it is smooth slowly add the grated Romano.

Add garlic, spinach, and chopped artichokes to the cream cheese. Once kind of combined add the mozzarella and Romano, once combined add the warmed alfredo.

You can refrigerate at this point, you want to serve this warm. So, timing for me is key!

When you are ready to bake it, you will bake it at 350 degrees for about 45 minutes to 1 hour.

Stuffed Peppers

9 Hungarian peppers
1/4 cup panko crumbs
7 oz. Parmesan, Fontina, Provolone, Asiago blend
Italian seasoning

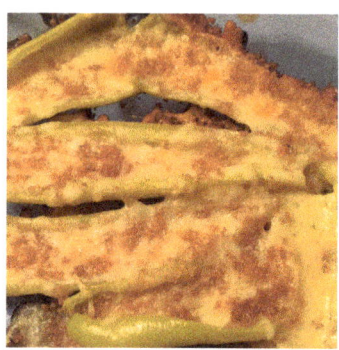

Wash peppers, if not organic wash in a vinegar bath. Cut lengthwise and if you don't want them very spicy make sure to deseed thoroughly.

Once peppers are prepped, lay flat in a Pyrex pie dish. Place them very close and add panko to the inside. There is no measuring here you just want a little layer on the bottom of the pepper and now you will stuff it with the 4-cheese blend that is pregrated.

You can use any cheese blend but this one is incredible for these peppers. You will top the peppers with more panko and the Italian seasonings.

Bake at 400 degrees about 10–15 minutes, until cheese is melted. Once they are done I put them on a plate and cut them in 1/4-inch slices.

Swiss Chard Pizza

1 bakery pizza dough
3 cups Swiss chard, chopped
1 cup broccoli, chopped
1/2 cup red pepper, diced
2 1/2–3 cups mozzarella

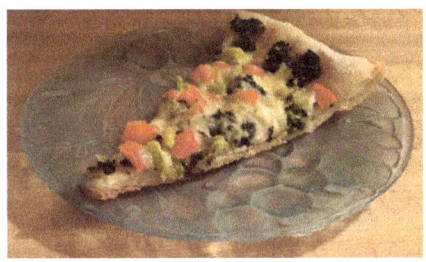

Preheat your pizza stone in an oven of 400 degrees for 20 minutes, I do this while I am prepping my pizzas.

Spread out your dough on the pizza stone and cover the whole pizza with the Swiss chard, and then layer the broccoli, and another layer of the red peppers. Now you can add the Mozzarella on top before putting it in the oven.

Cook your pizza for 20 minutes or until cheese is melted and crust is browned.

You can use kale or spinach instead. Also, if the greens are out of season you can use frozen.

Vegetable Pizza

1 bakery pizza dough
1 cup tomato sauce
1/2 cup spinach, chopped
1/2 cup broccoli, chopped
1/4 cup carrots, chopped
1/2 cup black olives, sliced
1/4 cup onions, sliced
5 oz. fresh Mozzarella, diced

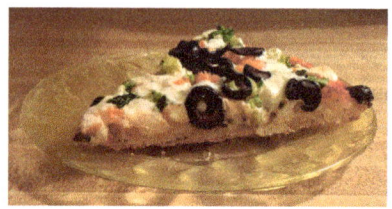

Preheat your pizza stone in an oven of 400 degrees for 20 minutes, I do this while I am prepping my pizzas.

Chop all ingredients, I use plain tomato sauce, nothing is added only tomatoes, I then add a tablespoon of Italian seasonings.

Coat dough with your sauce and add all of the vegetables, they will cook thoroughly. Add mozzarella evenly on top. Add black olives last, I love onions but my daughter doesn't so I add the onions only on 1/2 of our pizza.

Cook your pizza for 20 minutes or until cheese is melted and crust is browned.

Be creative, if you like different vegetables then do try them out!

White Pizza

1 bakery pizza dough
2 vine ripe tomatoes, sliced
2–3 cloves garlic, diced fine
2 cups mozzarella, shredded

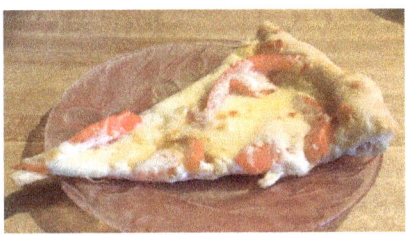

Preheat your pizza stone in an oven of 400 degrees for 20 minutes, I do this while I am prepping my pizzas.

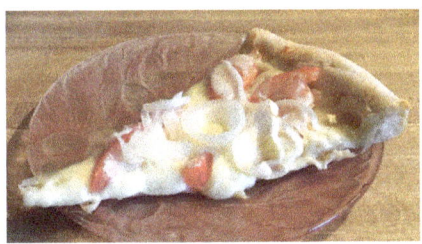

Slice your tomatoes and if you are using onions slice them also. Spread out your dough on the pizza stone and cover the whole pizza with the garlic and the tomatoes. Now add your mozzarella on top. If using onions, I put them on top of the cheese.

Cook your pizza for 20 minutes or until cheese is melted and crust is browned.

Remember, every stove is different, at the 15–20 minute mark check your pizza if it needs a few extra minutes that's okay!

Zakuska

2 onions, 3 1/2 cups
1 12 oz. jar fire roasted red
  peppers, 6 peppers
2 medium eggplants or 1 large
1 28 oz. can crushed tomatoes
2 tbsp. olive oil

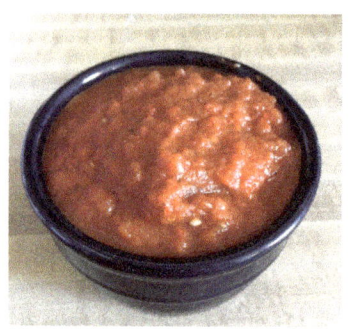

Preheat oven to 350 degrees, make slits in your eggplant, bake on a baking sheet for 30 minutes. Meanwhile, rough chop the onions and the peppers, sauté the onions in the olive oil about 10 minutes before adding the peppers. Stir often and sauté an additional 10 minutes, remove eggplant from the oven.

You will notice the skin already peeling away, once cooled peel the rest of the skin off and trim the top and bottom off. Slice your eggplant in half the long way and continue to slice it into 8 slices. Now cube those slices and add them to the onions and peppers. Sauté an additional 5 minutes, and add the crushed tomatoes. Stir and cook till it is slightly boiling. Shut the heat off and allow to cool before you will puree the mixture in a food processor in small batches.

Once pureed, it will be slightly chunky. Serve with pita or vegetables.

I prefer a crushed tomato with basil, and I also use my rosemary bread as a companion to this dish.

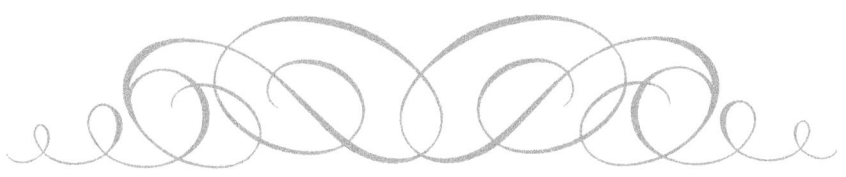

Desserts

You have *received* without paying, so *give* without being paid.

—Matthew 10:8

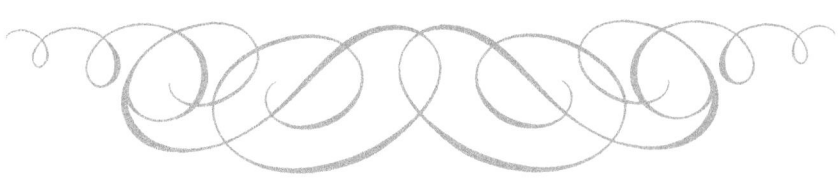

So now the section I am sure most of you did not think would be included in my book—desserts!

Now this is a section that my daughter wants to take off my hands, she says, "Mom, you are the cook and I am the baker." And she's right, if it were up to me I really wouldn't make desserts, they are not my favorite. But everyone I know loves a really good dessert and she is really getting good at it! Trying recipes I wouldn't have thought of but like me, she is figuring out the healthier way to make them.

I love watching her! I have to admit it is very hard to stay out of the kitchen though! I am very used to being the soul cook in my household, but really enjoy watching her become a cook like her mom. She researches recipes, we talk about ingredients and then we test them out. I have always been afraid of baking, I always had this idea that you have to follow a recipe to a tee and never falter from it or it will be a disaster. Maybe that is why I haven't made many attempts in this area. But I am so glad that this has been totally wrong, in seeing the recipes she wants to try and using the ingredients I would rather her use, we have both been pleasantly surprised with everything she has made!

But those are her recipes, so here you will find my recipes that I make for her birthday parties or at holiday times.

Apple Crisp

4 large apples
1/3 cup raw honey
2 tbs. garbanzo bean flour
1 tbs. lemon juice
1/2 tsp. ground cinnamon

Topping

1 cup old-fashioned oats
1/2 cup garbanzo bean flour
1/2 cup almonds or pecans
1/3 cup brown sugar
4 tbs. butter
3 tbs. Greek yogurt

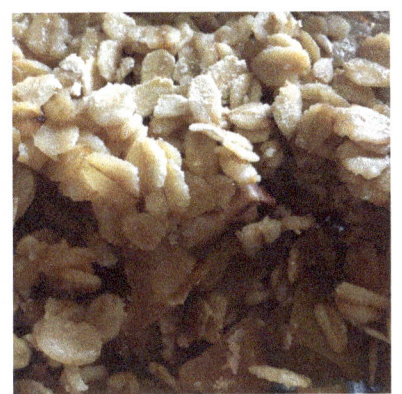

Preheat oven to 350 degrees. In one bowl mix the apples, honey, flour, lemon juice, and cinnamon. Mix together.

In another bowl mix the oats, flour, chopped nuts if you desire them, I do recommend them! Brown sugar, melted butter, and Greek yogurt. Stir until everything is combined and moistened.

In a 9x9" or 9x13" Pyrex pan coat with coconut oil and add your apple mixture, now add the oat mixture to the top and spread evenly. Bake for about 45–50 minutes or until the filling is bubbling on the edges and the top is a golden color.

Let it rest 5–10 minutes before serving.

If I have made Caramel, I will drizzle it on the top and bake an extra 5 minutes before cooling.

Apple Sauce

4 apples or 4 cups
1/2 tbs. cinnamon, nutmeg,
chia Seasoning
3 tbs. water

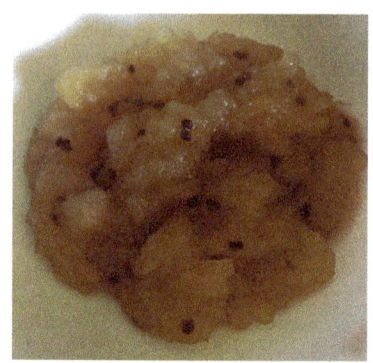

    Peel and cut apples in small chunks and add to a pot with the water and seasonings. Simmer on low heat covered and stir occasionally. After about 15 minutes the apples will be softened enough and ready to hand mash into applesauce. Once mashed and heat is off cover for 5 more minutes and mash one more time before serving.
    A regular sized apple is a cup.
    I use gala apples for this recipe.
    Don't be surprised if this doesn't last long, you can double the recipe or store it in the refrigerator for later use, but use within a week.
    If you cannot find this blend of seasonings, you can blend them yourself.

Beet Brownies

2 medium beets, roasted
1 cup unsweetened almond milk
1 tsp. apple cider vinegar
3/4 cup organic sugar
1/4 cup coconut oil
2 tsp. pure vanilla extract
1 cup and 1 tbsp. garbanzo bean flour
1/2 cup 100% pure cocoa powder
1 tsp. baking soda
1/2 tsp. baking powder
1/2 cup mini chocolate chips

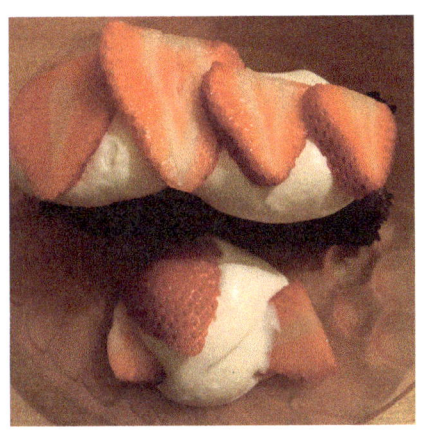

Once your beets are cooled, finely grate on a cheese grater, measure out 1/2 cup and set aside.

You can either line muffin pans with paper liners or make as a brownie cake in a glass pan. I use a Pyrex 7x11" pan and coat it with coconut oil. Preheat oven to 375 degrees.

Whisk together the almond milk and vinegar in a large bowl and set aside a few minutes to allow to curdle. Add the sugar, oil, vanilla, and 1/2 cup beets and beat until foamy. No need to melt coconut oil as it will harden in this mixture just mix as well as you can. Add the garbanzo bean flour, 100% pure unsweetened cocoa powder, baking soda, baking powder, and mini chips, mix well either by hand or with a mixer.

Pour batter into liners 3/4 full, or all into the pan, bake 25 minutes or until toothpick comes out clean. Store in an airtight container to stay fresh.

Caramel Apple Nachos

1/2 cup sugar
2 tbs. water
1/2 tbs. lemon juice
1 cup coconut milk, full fat
1 tsp. vanilla
6–8 apples
1 tbs. lemon juice
1 handful of chocolate chips

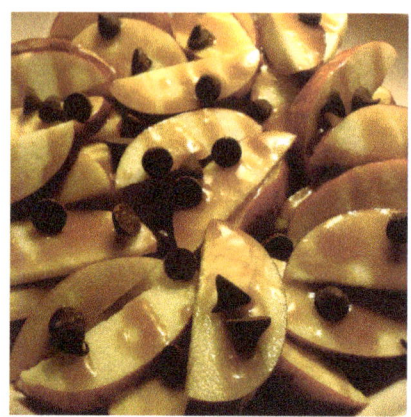

In a small pot over medium low heat, mix sugar, water, and lemon juice to a boil, stirring constantly so the mixture won't burn.

Once boiling, pour coconut milk slowly and add vanilla while mixing. Simmer for about 15 minutes until mixture becomes darker and thickens. Be sure to stir occasionally and scrape the sides of your pan to avoid burning. Remove from heat once thick and cool down to room temperature.

Prepare your apples in slices, and mix with lemon juice to avoid browning once caramel is done drizzle on apple slices and top with chocolate chips.

For best results store in a sealed jar overnight in refrigerator before using.

I use this caramel for my ice cream creations too!

Cheesecake Bites

3–8 oz. cream cheese
1 1/4 cup sugar, divided
5 eggs
1 3/4 tsp. vanilla, divided
1 cup sour cream
2 tbsp. jam
fresh berries

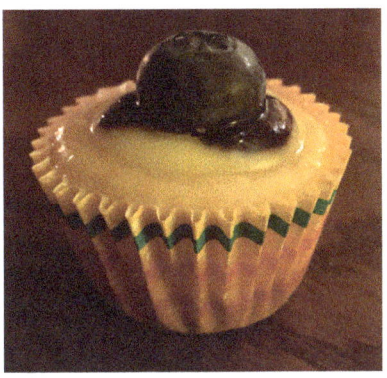

    Beat the cream cheese with 1 cup sugar and eggs in a large bowl. Add 1 1/2 tsp. vanilla. Pour batter into paper liners, filling 2/3 full. Bake for 40 minutes.

    Combine sour cream, 1/4 cup sugar, and 1/4 tsp. vanilla and mix well.

    Remove cupcakes from oven when done. They will fall in the middle, fill fallen center with sour cream mixture. Spoon 1/4 tsp. jam on top of each and return to the oven and bake for 5 minutes.

    Garnish with fresh berries.

Chocolate Chick Bars

2 14 oz. cans chick peas
1 cup almond butter
2/3 cup maple syrup
2 tbsp. vanilla extract
1/2 tsp. sea salt
1/2 tsp. baking soda
1/2 tsp. baking powder
2/3 cup chocolate chips

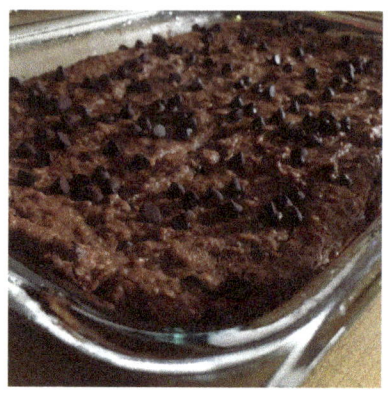

    Preheat the oven to 350 degrees. Coat a 9x13" glass baking dish with coconut oil. In a food processor, combine the drained chickpeas, almond butter, maple syrup, extract, salt, baking soda, and baking powder. Blend until smooth. Add some of the chocolate chips to the mixture and save some to add to the top. Bake 40–50 minutes or until the edges are golden and a toothpick comes out clean. Remove and let cool at least 20 minutes.

    This recipe is doubled if you would just like to make a smaller batch cut the recipe in half and use a loaf pan. Either way they come out delicious!

Cinnamon Sugar Almonds

1 egg white
1 tsp. water
4 cups whole raw almonds
1/2 cup sugar
1/4 tsp. salt
1/2 tsp. ground cinnamon

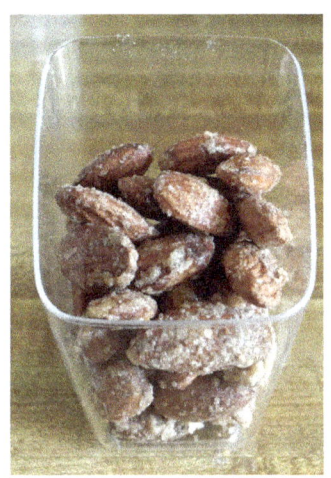

Preheat oven to 250 degrees, and bake on a parchment paper lined cookie sheet.

Beat egg white and water till frothy and add nuts. Mix to coat, once completely coated add mixed sugar, salt and cinnamon over the nuts and again mix till thoroughly combined and coated.

Lay in one layer on lined cookie sheet and bake for 1 hour, you will need to check them often and toss every 5–10 minutes. Break apart if they start to stick.

After one hour, pull out of oven and cool on top of oven for half an hour. They will crisp as they cool. Once cooled, store in an airtight container.

These nuts make great gifts and are perfect for the little snack.

Cinnamon Tortillas

1 pkg. flour tortillas
1/2 cup sugar
2 tbsp. cinnamon
water

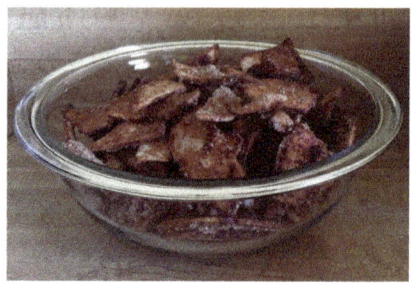

Cut tortillas in wedges, depending on the size tortillas you buy this may vary. A small tortilla I would cut in eight. But a large tortilla I would try to get 16–20 chips out of it. I use a pizza cutter to make cutting easier.

Once cut, spray or dip all wedges in water and combine sugar and cinnamon either in a container with a lid or a gallon ziplock bag.

Add wet tortillas to the sugar mix, close and shake vigorously till coated.

Heat oven to 400 and add tortilla wedges to an olive or coconut oil pan. Bake till light brown and crisp, about 6 minutes. Check 1/2 way to see if you should flip.

1 package of small tortilla shells I had 2 cookie sheets full of tortillas.

Cookie Dough Balls

1 stick butter, softened
3/4 cup brown sugar
2 tsps. vanilla
1/2 tsp. salt
1 cup all-purpose flour
2 tbsps. almond milk
1/2 cup mini chocolate chips

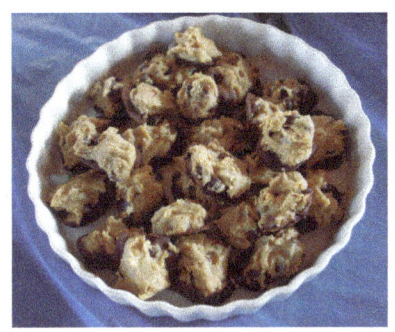

Cream butter and brown sugar, add vanilla and salt, mix. Add in flour, mixture should be crumbly. Add in the almond milk and mix thoroughly. Now it will look like cookie dough, fold in the chocolate chips.

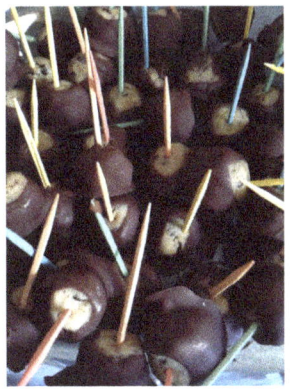

Make mini balls and freeze, the next day melt chocolate chips or dark chocolate and dip each mini ball.

Refreeze till you are ready to serve.

I make these for birthday parties and they do not last, you may want to make 2 batches or more.

Fruit Salsa

1–2 Granny Smith apples
8 strawberries
3 kiwis
1 tsp. cinnamon
1/2 tsp. vanilla

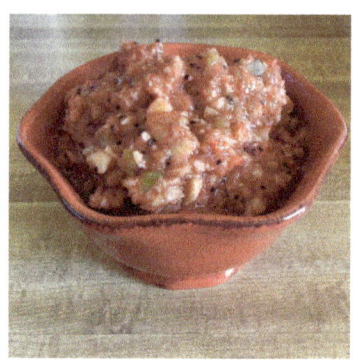

Core apples, hull strawberries, and peel kiwis. Cut all fruit in smaller pieces and add to food processor with the cinnamon and vanilla.

Pulse in food processor till fully combined. Serve with Cinnamon Tortillas.

Hot Fudge

2 cups chocolate chips
1 cup coconut milk, can
1/4 cup raw honey
1 tsp. vanilla

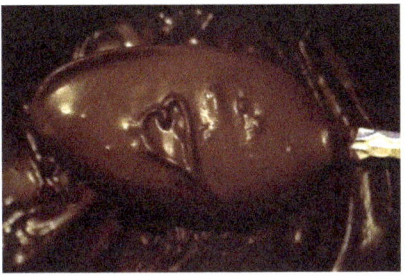

Add all ingredients to a small pan that is in a wider pan with water, a double boiler. Heat on medium low and stir constantly until the mixture becomes silky smooth, about 5–10 minutes.

I add this as a middle layer to my ice cream cakes but can be used as a topping for ice cream also.

Please check my website for the ingredients I use.

Ice Cream

1 cup almond milk
1/2 cup sugar
2 cups heavy cream
1–2 tsp. vanilla extract

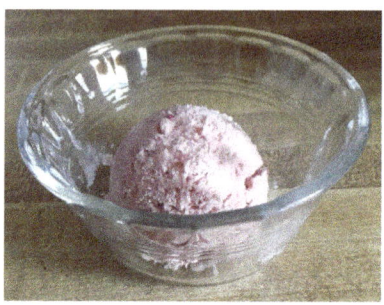

This is the base for all of my ice creams, and yes, I make a lot of flavors. I use an ice cream maker, so I will blend all of these ingredients by hand until I can tell the sugar has combined and melted into the creams, you do not want to see the sugar when you add it to the machine. Every machine is different mine takes about 15–20 minutes to combine and will stiffen up more when in the freezer.

The picture above is my cherry ice cream, I rough chop a 1/2 cup or more of farm fresh frozen cherries and I add them after the ice cream is starting to take form.

Everyone loves cookie dough! This recipe I make my Cookie Dough Ball recipe and make mini balls and add them to the ice cream once it is finished in the machine. If you add them to the machine they may clog it, just fold them in after.

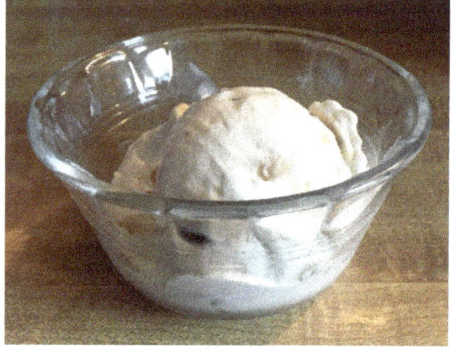

Ice Cream Cakes

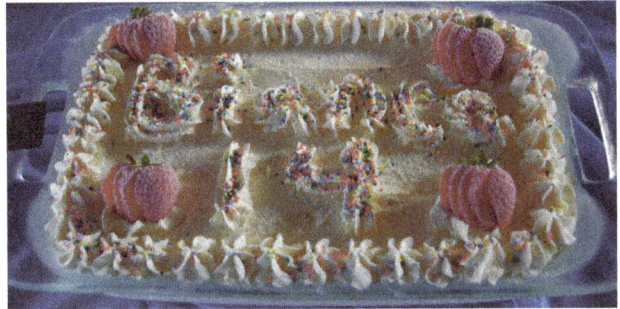

I only make ice cream cakes for birthdays, and these have got to be my most favorite desserts to make. I always make them the way the birthday girl wants them made.

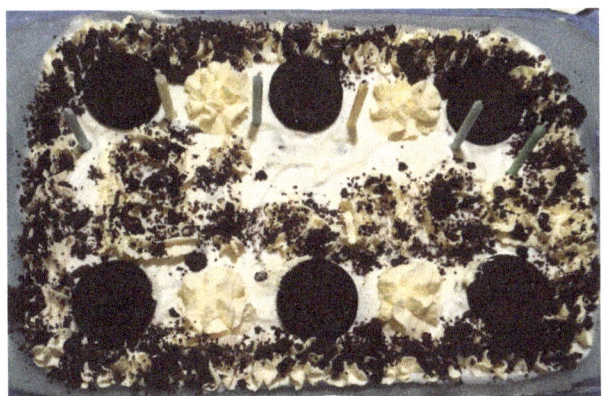

They always start with my basic Ice Cream recipe, and there is always a vanilla layer and then a layer of the birthday girl's choice. In the top picture it was vanilla and strawberry, and the middle was a cookie crumb with my Caramel Sauce. For decorating the top I always use our homemade Whip Cream.

The second cake was a vanilla layer and a chocolate layer, and the middle was a chocolate cookie crumb with our homemade Fudge Sauce. The decorated topping is always our homemade Whip Cream and this one needed more cookie crumbs.

Pumpkin Dip

16 oz. organic cottage cheese
1 cup organic pure pumpkin puree
1 tsp. apple cider vinegar
2 tsps. pumpkin pie spice
2 tsps. cinnamon

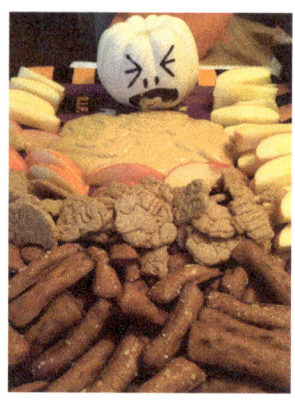

Place all ingredients in blender or food processor and puree until very smooth.

Refrigerate for later or serve immediately. Pairs well with apples!

As you can see I make this one for Halloween!

Rhubarb Bread

2 cups garbanzo bean flour
1/2 cup sugar
1 tbsp. baking powder
3/4 cup almond milk
3 tbsps. coconut oil
1 egg, beaten
1 cup rhubarb, finely chopped
1 tsp. orange zest

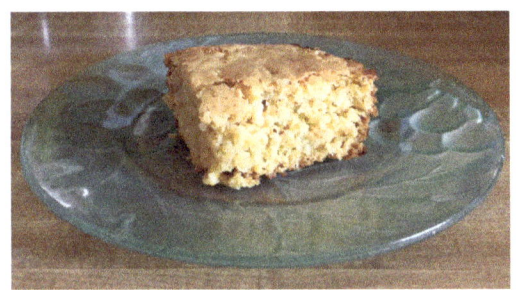

 Preheat oven to 400 degrees. Prepare a 9x13" glass baking dish with coconut oil. Mix all dry ingredients in a separate bowl. Blend the wet ingredients well adding the coconut oil last, this will not blend in perfectly and will clump but it will be fine once baked. Stir in the rhubarb and the orange zest into the dry ingredient bowl. Once combined, add the dry ingredients to the wet and mix well. Pour into prepared baking dish and bake for 18–23 minutes. Cool for 15 minutes before cutting and serving.

 This is one you will be surprised with as was I. It has the texture of a cornbread but a taste that will have you coming back for more.

 As you can imagine, I do cut the sugar back on this one a bit, too, make it and use your judgment with your second batch.

Spicy Almonds

1 egg white
1 tsp. water
4 cups raw whole almonds
1/4 cup sugar
1 tsp. salt
1 tsp. paprika
1 tsp. garlic powder
1 tsp. onion powder
1/4 tsp. black pepper
1/4 tsp. cayenne pepper

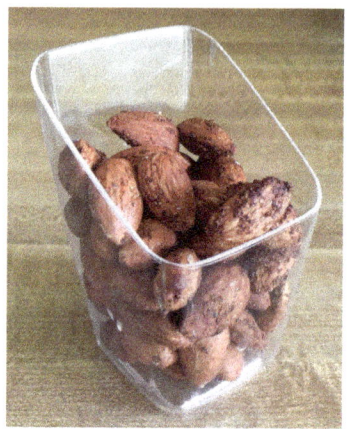

Preheat oven to 275 degrees, and bake on a parchment paper lined cookie sheet.

Beat egg white and water till frothy and add nuts. Mix to coat.

In a small bowl, combine all of the spices and add to the nuts, stir to combine.

Lay in one layer on lined cookie sheet and bake for 45 minutes, you will need to check them often and toss every 5–10 minutes. Break apart if they start to stick.

Pull out of oven and cool on top of oven for half an hour. They will crisp as they cool.

Strawberry Rhubarb Crumble

4 cups fresh rhubarb, chopped
1 pint strawberries, sliced
1 tbsp. honey
1/2 cup brown sugar
1/4 cup butter
1 tsp. ground cinnamon
1 cup oats

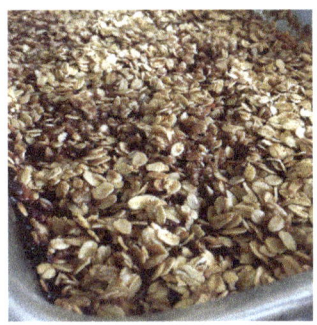

Preheat the oven to 350 degrees. Chop and peel the rhubarb and hull and slice the strawberries. In a medium bowl, stir the honey into the rhubarb and strawberries.

Use coconut oil to grease a 9x13" Pyrex glass baking dish and place your fruit mixture into it. In the same bowl, stir together the oats, brown sugar (I use less), and cinnamon. Mix in the butter until it is crumbly, and spread over the top of the fruit.

Bake for 40 minutes, until rhubarb is tender and the topping is toasted.

Serve warm.

Depending on the strawberries, I will use up to a pound. Mix yours and see if you want to add more!

Always yummy topped with my Whip Cream recipe!

Watermelon Cake

whole watermelon
Whip Cream
blueberries to decorate

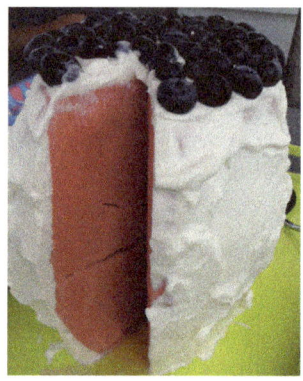

Any size of watermelon works, of course I buy organic fruit and have used mini watermelons and large watermelons.

Depending on the size and how you carve the rind, your watermelon can stand up like the one pictured or lay down.

Use the recipe for the whip cream and use a spatula to spread the whip cream on your watermelon.

You can use any other fruit to decorate your watermelon cake. I have done them many different ways. The way I have pictured is basic, but you can get as creative as you would like!

Whip Cream

1 pint or 2 cups heavy cream
1 tbs. powdered sugar
1 tsp. vanilla

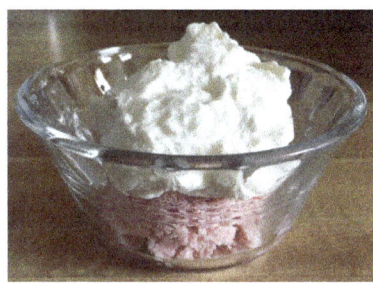

    Add all ingredients to a mixing bowl, when measuring the powdered sugar, do not level your spoon, you want it to heap over a little bit.

    We only hand whip our whip cream, yes it is more of a job, but it comes out so much better when you add this extra love to it.

    You will know when it is done, you will whip it about 5 minutes or so with a whisk but it will feel like hours to your hand. This is a great hand workout. You will see it form into whip cream and the taste is unlike any other whip cream you may have had! You will not mind making this one over and over again!

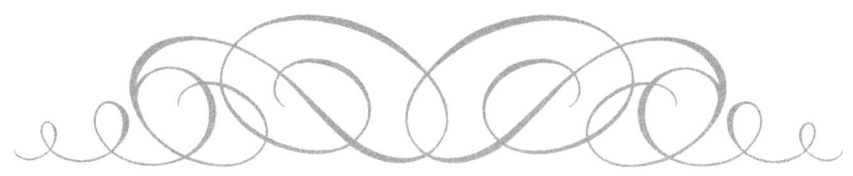

Cravings

No one experiencing temptation should say, "I am being tempted by God," for God is not subject to temptation to evil, and he himself tempts no one. Rather each person is tempted when he is lured and enticed by his own desire.

—James 1:13–14

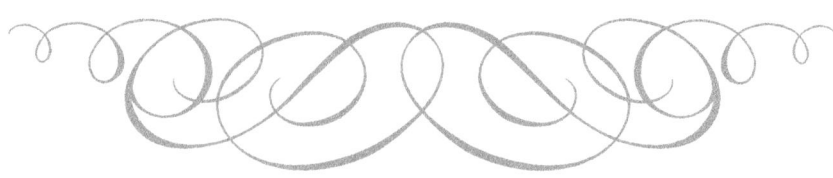

LIVE NATURALLY

Have you ever wondered why out of nowhere sometimes you crave things? It comes on quickly with no warning like an uncontrollable urge, usually for a specific food and nothing else can take its place. The cravings almost always are for something not healthy and definitely not good for you. Food cravings may actually be your body's way of telling you it is lacking key nutrients. You may think cravings are weaknesses but they are not. The reason why we tend to think of unhealthy food is because of what we have been marketed most of our lives, it is time to change our thoughts and find what we really should be eating instead.

I have created a list of the most common cravings and what nutrients your body may be lacking:

- acidic foods – magnesium
- alcohol – protein, avenin, calcium, and/or potassium
- bread, pasta, and other carbs – nitrogen
- burnt food – carbon
- chocolate – magnesium
- chewing ice – iron
- coffee or tea – phosphorus, sulfur, NaC1 (salt), and/or iron
- cool drinks – manganese
- lack of appetite – vitamin B1, vitamin B3, manganese, and/or chloride
- liquids rather than solids – water
- oily foods – calcium
- overeating – silicon, tryptophan, and/or tyrosine
- soda and carbonated drinks – calcium
- premenstrual or menopausal cravings – zinc
- salty foods – chloride
- solids rather than liquids – water
- sweets – chromium, carbon, phosphorus, sulfur, and/or tryptophan

Here are some healthier alternatives to have when our bodies are craving these foods:

- avenin – granola, oatmeal (not if you have celiac disease)
- calcium – legumes, cheese, sesame, broccoli, kale, mustard, and turnip greens
- carbon – fresh fruits
- chloride – raw goat milk, fatty fish, and unrefined salt
- chromium – broccoli, grapes, cheese, dried beans, chicken, calf's liver
- iron – meat, fish, poultry, seaweed, greens, black cherries
- manganese – walnuts, almonds, pecans, pineapple, blueberries
- magnesium – fruits, legumes, raw cacao, raw nuts, and seeds
- NaCl (salt) – sea salt, apple cider vinegar
- nitrogen – high protein foods like fish, meats, nuts, and beans
- phosphorous – chicken, beef, liver, poultry, fish, eggs, dairy, nuts, legumes, grains
- potassium – bitter greens, seaweed, sundried black olives, potato peel broth
- protein – meat, poultry, seafood, dairy, nuts
- silicon – seeds, nuts, (avoid refined starches)
- sulfur – kale, cabbage, garlic, red peppers, onion, cruciferous vegetables, horseradish, cranberries, egg yolks
- tryptophan – cheese, liver, lamb, raisins, sweet potato, spinach
- tyrosine – red, orange and green fruits and vegetables
- vitamin B1 – nuts, seeds, beans, liver, and other organ meats
- vitamin B3 – tuna, halibut, beef, chicken, turkey, pork, seeds, legumes
- zinc – leafy vegetables, root vegetables, seafood

A lot of times when you have been dehydrated for so long you no longer thirst. A healthier alternative to water if you have trouble drinking, is to add lemon or lime to your water.

This is an awful lot to think about, I myself have read this so many times over the years and still in that moment of your cravings it may be hard to remember what your body actually needs versus what you think you want.

When you eat a nutritionally dense, well-balanced diet, you may find you no longer have cravings for sweet and salty foods. It makes sense that a diet full of the necessary vitamins and minerals will prevent cravings. But in our fast-paced society this may seem next to impossible. It doesn't have to be, baby steps one change at a time brings you closer to a healthier you!

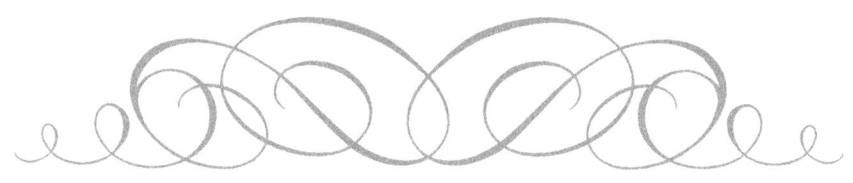

Knowledge Is Power

God also said, "See, I give you every
seed-bearing plant all over the earth and
every tree that has seed-bearing fruit on
it to be your food; and to all the animals of the
land, all the birds of the air, and all
living creatures that crawl on the ground,
I give all the green plants for food." And
so it happened.

—Genesis 1:29–30

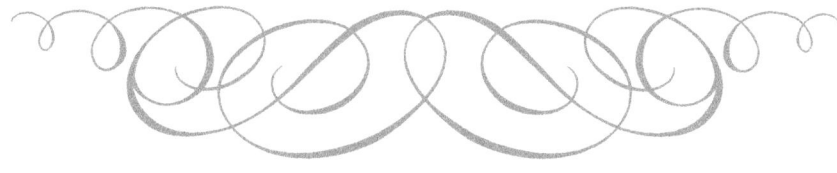

This is not my information, this information has been in existence forever, but I, as maybe others, have lost sight of it or may never have made the connection.

I am including it because sometimes I need to refer to it and some of this has become some of my most valuable information. I believe it is important to pass along and share it with others.

Have you ever wondered why things look like other things?

There are many signs in this life we just have to be open to them—plants, trees, vegetables, and fruits that were created by God for a purpose to feed us and to help heal us naturally.

Some examples with food are very well known, take for example:

- Beans – help heal and maintain kidney function and I bet it is not a coincidence one bean was named after this organ just for looks.

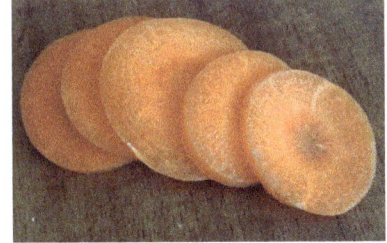

- Carrots – they enhance blood flow to the eyes and when sliced, look like the eye.

- Ginger – it is no wonder ginger aids in digestion, it looks like the stomach. Did you know it also could cure nausea and motion sickness? There is research showing it can slow down the growth of bowel tumors also.

- Tomatoes – have four chambers and are red just like the heart. What is the best food for our heart? Lycopene and guess what tomatoes are full of!

- Walnuts – what does a walnut look like to you? Yes, a brain! Well, did you know that walnuts help develop neurotransmitters to enhance brain function.
  Something a little less known maybe.

- Avocados, eggplants, and pears – this one I wish I knew about years ago, but am glad I do now and another good reason I was eating all the eggplant I was when I was pregnant. These wonderful foods are good for the health of the womb and the cervix and look just like these organs. Research has now shown that if a woman eats one avocado a week it balances birth hormones, sheds unwanted birth weight, and can even prevent cervical cancer. It takes an avocado nine months to grow from blossom to ripened fruit, coincidence? I think not.

- Bananas – did you know bananas contain a protein called tryptophan and when we digest it, it converts to a neurotransmitter called serotonin which is a mood regulating chemical in the brain, is that why a banana looks like a smile?

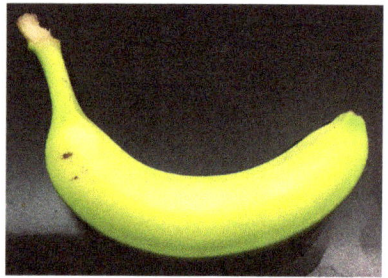

One of my students loves bananas and gets so excited when he sees them for his breakfast or his lunch. It is an extra special day if they are offered at both breakfast and lunch, and he always says to me, "Oh, goody! How I love bananas!" This to me explains it perfectly, through the eyes of this innocent child!

- Celery, bok choy, and rhubarb – did you think they would be in the same family? Well, these are foods that specifically target bone strength. Bones are 23% sodium and these foods are 23% sodium. If you do not have enough sodium in your diet, the body pulls it from your bones and makes them weak, and don't they look like bones?

- Citrus Fruits – look like mammary glands of the female breast and assist the health of the breast and lymph nodes.

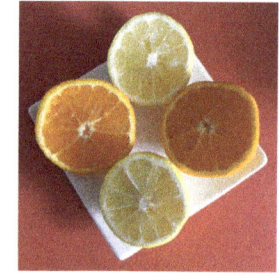

- Figs – are full of seeds and hang in twos when they grow. I'm sure you see where I am going with this one. Studies show figs increase mobility of male sperm and increase sperm count as well as overcoming male sterility.

- Grapes – look like blood cells and the more research that has been done shows they are great for the heart and blood, but they also help boost the immune system and helps cure asthma and migraines. They have so many benefits to help your overall health!

- Mushrooms – when sliced in half, what do you think a mushroom looks like? That's right, a human ear. Some research has shown that mushrooms can improve hearing since they contain vitamin D which is healthy for bones especially the three tiny bones in the ear that transmit sound to the brain.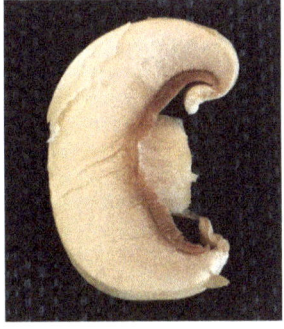

- Olives – assist the health and function of ovaries. It has been shown that women who have diets high in olive oil have lower risks of ovarian cancer. For optimal benefits make sure your olive oil is extra virgin organic cold pressed olive oil.

- Onions – did you ever wonder why onions make you cry? Do you not like onions because of this? Actually, you should thank onions for this odd reaction for they are actually helping you wash the epithelial layers of the eyes. They also help clear waste materials from all of the body's cells.

- Sweet potatoes – look like the pancreas so it should be no surprise they actually balance the glycemic index of diabetics.

Again, this is not my information, if you have had any of these ailments, I suggest you try them and continue your own research on them—knowledge is power! We do need to take control of our own health!

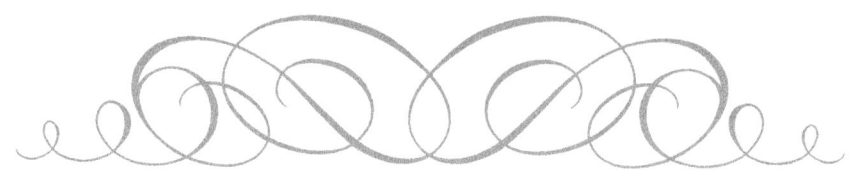

Water

God can restore what is broken and change it into something amazing. All you need is *Faith*.

—Joel 2:25

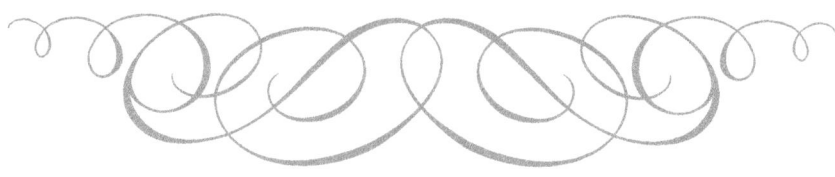

Now that I have shared all of my go-to food recipes I feel it is time to talk about whole body wellness and how to keep you and your family as healthy as possible. And I think I need to share with you some of my go-to home remedies to put to use before, during, and after an illness.

First up, water!

We are made up mostly of water, yet for some reason, this is extremely hard for a lot of people to drink during their day. But we can drink a 16 oz. pop, or a 20 oz. coffee, or even a 12 oz. beer, no problem. And let's be real, these drinks we can usually drink more than one of. It truly does come down to a mindset, if you have your mind set on getting healthy, it is easier to drink water than you may think it is.

So let's think about water for a second, what do you think of it? Do you like it, can you not drink it at all, do you worry about our water and aren't sure how to get the purest water?

There are so many different theories to how much water a person should have each day. The magic number we have all heard is 8–8 oz. of glasses a day. Well, that is 64 oz. a day. Now, if you exercise, the magic number is 1/2 your body weight in ounces. Let's look at it this way, the human body is anywhere from 55–78% water depending on body size.

Muscle consists of 75% water.
Brain consists of 90% water.
Bone consists of 22% water.
Blood consists of 83% water!

Every cell in your body needs water. For example, your brain consists of 90% water, if you don't supply enough water to your body your brain can't function well, and you will get a headache or migraine. Harmful effects and symptoms of dehydration are fatigue, migraine, constipation, dark urine, muscle cramps, irregular blood pressure, kidney problems, dry skin, thirst, hunger, and if 20% dehydrated, a risk of death.

So how much water should you drink a day? There is not a magic number. Everyone is different, it depends on your health condition, your activity level, your physical size, your weight, and your environment. Spread your water out evenly throughout the day.

When you wake up drink a glass of water to get your body ready for the day, it helps activate your internal organs. A few hours later drink a glass of water with lemon and if you really want to add extra health benefits to your water add apple cider vinegar! Drink a glass of water a 1/2 an hour before a meal, it helps digestion. During your meal, try not to drink as it flushes the nutrients from your meal too quickly through your system and some nutrients may be lost. Always drink water before, during, and after exercise. You need your muscles to be lubricated and ready to be flexible. Again, always drink a glass of water before a shower it helps lower your blood pressure, it also decreases your risk of passing out from the heat of the shower. A glass of water before bed helps your body avoid a stroke or a heart attack.

I have a lot of theories when it comes to drinking water, as you can see. But I am very particular on drinking water when we wake in the morning and here is why. When we wake up and drink a glass of water, it helps activate our internal organs. Water balances your lymph system, these glands help you perform daily functions, balance your body fluids, and fight infection. Drinking water on an empty stomach also purifies the colon making it easier to absorb nutrients. It also increases the production of new blood and muscle cells. Water also helps to purge toxins from the blood which helps keep your skin glowing and clear. Drinking at least 16 oz. of chilled water can boost your metabolism by 24% in the morning. Something so simple can do your body so much good! And all of this even before you leave your house in the morning!

So now that I have shared with you some of the facts about water I will share with you what I do on a daily basis.

When I wake up I pour 25 oz. of water with a shot of lemon juice and a shot of apple cider vinegar, I say a shot because I do not measure, I shake them and pour them as I am getting my water from my fridge. My fridge has a water dispenser that is filtered, this is my main source of water throughout my day. About 3 hours later, I will make my protein shake, which again is mostly water. I drink 2 25 oz. cups of water in the morning prior to lunch and I do not drink with my lunch. As you see, this is already more than 1/2 my body weight in ounces, so you may think this is too much but for me, because I exercise and walk a lot throughout my day, this is perfect for me and it is something that I worked up to. If you are not a water drinker you need to add water to your daily routine slowly, I would start with a glass upon rising and try to stick to these theories but don't drink as much and every few weeks add a few more ounces to each serving throughout your day.

Listen to your body, it does tell you when it is thirsty. Pay attention to your hair, skin, mouth, and eyes. When you start adding more water you will notice these parts of your body improving. Not so hard, right? Now tell me, how much water do you drink a day?

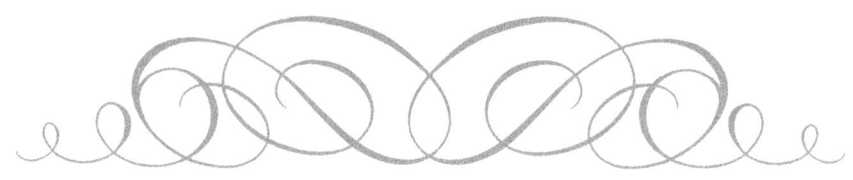

Apple Cider Vinegar

Beloved, I hope you are prospering in every respect and are in good health, just as your soul is prospering.

—3 John 1:2

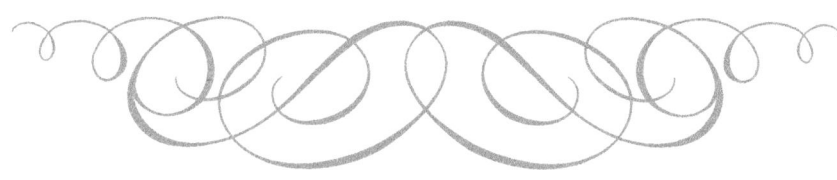

It's not a secret, my love for apple cider vinegar. Raw apple cider vinegar is the only vinegar we want to consume. It is non-acid forming and is great in salad dressing. When purchasing apple cider vinegar, make sure you purchase raw, organic, unfiltered, unpasteurized, and has the mother intact apple cider vinegar. The mother is the buildup of yeast and bacteria that builds up during the slow fermentation process. It is commonly thought to contain most of the beneficial enzymes and proteins. The mother makes apple cider vinegar look cloudy and may even have strands or sediment in the bottom of your apple cider vinegar. This is what you want, make sure you shake it well to disperse the mother before you use it.

Apple cider vinegar is known to contain vitamins like magnesium and B6 that you need to keep your body healthy. It also contains minerals, amino acids, and acetic acid, which has the ability to kill bad bacteria and grow good bacteria, it acts as a natural antibiotic. Apple cider vinegar is also known to contain polyphenolic compounds, which are known for their role in preventing disease. Because apple cider vinegar is made from apples it contains pectin. Pectin acts as a prebiotic that encourages a healthy gut by supporting the growth of probiotic bacteria.

Apple cider vinegar can be used for many things and can cure many ailments here are the most common uses for apple cider vinegar:

- detoxifies your body
- cures a cold
- lowers blood pressure
- balances blood sugar
- cures acid reflux and heartburn
- relieves allergies
- balances PH
- antifungal
- eases varicose veins
- soothes sunburn
- skin toner

- heals poison ivy
- removes warts
- candida cleanse
- weight loss aid
- repels fleas
- natural deodorant
- natural aftershave mixed with water
- hair conditioner
- whitens teeth
- relieves hiccups
- household cleaner that detoxifies your home
- all natural weed killer
- washes your fruits and vegetables of toxic sprays

As you see, you can use apple cider vinegar for many things. I also have used it on facial and neck blemishes and within a few applications have healed the skin.

This is the first thing I put in my body every day. I have already talked to you about water, so this is what I do to stay healthy.

My ACV Water

25 oz. water
1 tbsp. ACV
1 tbsp. lemon juice

I mix everything together and drink it within 5–10 minutes.

Do not drink apple cider vinegar straight, it can harm your esophagus. I don't sip it, but if you have a hard time, drink some and come back to it. You will get used to it!

This concoction helps my body wake up in the morning and get everything moving properly. I have worked at an elementary school in a k-1 special education class since 2010 and have never gotten sick. I have cleaned many runny noses, and many messy faces, and wiped many tears with overly loving hugs. If I feel something brewing, I double up and drink twice a day. Mind over matter is my rule and works for me!

My family will tell you I like the taste, and that is not true but I know it works and they know it too. They don't drink it daily but they do drink my concoction when they feel a cold coming on and it keeps the cold or sore throat from getting any worse.

If you have not gone through all of my recipes you will see I do sneak it in to my cooking also.

Brussel Sprout Slaw
Kohlrabi Salad
Vinaigrette
Vegetable Pasta Salad
Beet Brownies
Pumpkin Dip

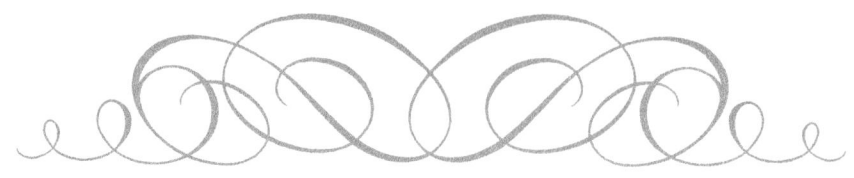

Kefir

Jesus looked at them and said,
"With man this is impossible
but with *God all things are possible.*"

—Matthew 19:26

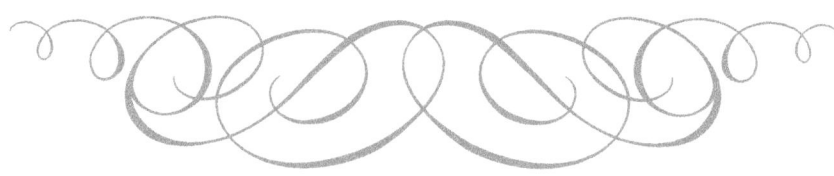

Now I will share with you my next home remedy for the times you haven't kept up on your ACV and you are starting to get sick.

First drink my ACV water now and make my Kefir Smoothie.

Kefir is known to:
ACV water
- regulate the immune system
- regulate cholesterol
- regulate sugar levels
- regulate blood pressure
- improve blood circulation
- strengthen the kidneys
- promote production of bile
- provide natural protection against disease
- slow down aging

It is excellent nourishment for everyone including children, pregnant and nursing moms, the elderly, and those with compromised immune systems.

Kefir is also known to:

- boost immunity
- build bone density
- improve lactose digestion
- heal inflammatory bowel disease
- fight allergies
- support detoxification.
- kefir can also help eliminate unhealthy food cravings by making the body more nourished and balanced.

There are many varieties of kefir, my suggestion is always buy plain. If you buy a flavor there is a lot of unneeded sugar added, you can follow my recipe or make your own to control the sugar content. Using the milk from cows, sheep, or goats makes kefir. But it can also be made by milk substitutes like rice milk, coconut milk, soymilk, coconut water, fruit juice, and ginger beer. Some may be harder to find than others but you can try many different versions to see what your family likes best. And if you know me you know I do not buy the soy version, but that is completely up to you and what your family prefers.

Do you need more reasons to make it a part of your daily routine?

As I said, this is my family's go-to on the rare occurrence of an illness, but we also drink it regularly to keep our bodies healthy since kefir is one of the highest probiotic foods you can eat, well, drink.

Please note if you have an allergy to dairy consult your physician first, or try kombucha, another favorite of ours!

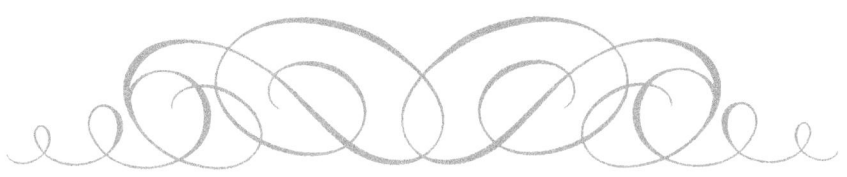

Headaches

Cast all of your worries upon *Him*,
because *He* cares for *You*.

—1 Peter 5:7

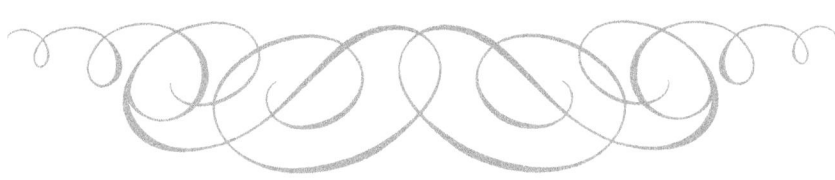

Now I have spoken to you at great lengths of my family's daily habits to keep us healthy at all times. But in cases where some ailments may pop up, I do have home remedies that I will tend to before we resort to modern-day medicine. I think it's a perfect time to share those with you so you can try them before reaching to your medicine cabinet.

We live in a world of now, we want to lose that stubborn last 10 pounds now and not bother to actually workout. We want to get to our destination now even though it literally is an hour drive. We have all seen the drivers, or sometimes we are one of them—weaving in and out of traffic just to get to the same red light as everyone else. We want relief from pain now and not allow the body time to heal.

We can never slow down, we must keep going.

When we have ailments it's our body's way of speaking to us trying to tell us what is wrong. But we are too much in a hurry to listen so we try to mask it instead of fix it.

So let's talk about headaches, I must admit I really have never had headaches except a few times as a teen. And I never knew much about migraines but I did know a few people that got them terribly and they would cause nosebleeds, or nearly cripple them for a few days where they could not leave their darkened rooms.

Well, up until my concussion I never thought I would have ever experienced them but on more than one occasion, I would have pain at the base of my neck that would shoot up to the top of my head toward my forehead. At night the lights on cars and streetlights would make my head spin and I could not focus let alone watch the road. After way too long of dealing with this, I mentioned it to my friend who was also my chiropractor. I never, in a million years, thought he could help me, to me it was a passing conversation but right away he explained to me that I was experiencing migraines and that he found a pinched nerve in my neck that through a series of adjustments over some time gave me relief. Yes, that concussion did a number on me but in the meantime it made me research and find natural things to help keep them at bay and I'm glad to say they have not returned.

So, headaches, did you know there are over 150 different types of headaches but 4 types that are the most common.

Tension or stress headaches can come and go over time and are mild to moderate usually.

Cluster headaches are more severe and occur in groups over about a week to a month's time. They may go away but can come back months to years later. They tend to occur more so behind the eyes.

Sinus headaches, now these can also be accompanied by other ailments like fever, runny nose, pressure in ears, pain in your cheeks, forehead, nose, and/or facial swelling. I have seen this happen to my dear friend and it is very painful.

Now migraines, these are different for everyone and can last an hour or a few days and may happen once a month or more. Usually people can have sensitivity to light, noises, or smells, loss of appetite, pain, nausea, or vomiting. You may feel dizzy, have blurred vision, or a fever. Wow, yeah, I had many of these at the same time.

A headache is another way of your body telling you something. So what is it telling you?

You may be lacking something like a vitamin or a nutrient deficiency, or food sensitivity. You may be lacking water or need to change the way you eat or you may just need to slow life down and take a breath.

Not many people like hearing these answers.

They also can be triggered by eyestrain, stress, fatigue, allergies, hormones, low blood sugar, constipation, drugs or alcohol, or poor posture—another reason to stand up straight. And yes, as I typed this I even sat up a bit straighter in my chair.

So I am sure you're wondering well what are the first things I should start with.

It will be hard to be patient when you are in pain, so try adapting this to your daily lifestyle to try to make it a bit easier. The first thing I am going to say is water, refer back to what I have already spoken about and try adding a bit more every day. Also, magnesium, it is the most successful and you can't over take it if your body has enough it will excrete it. You can get magnesium through foods like dark leafy vegetables, squashes, broccoli, whole grains, nuts and seeds, beans, dairy products, and meats. You can also get magnesium in dark chocolate and coffee. Okay, looking at that I can make a great dinner and dessert! But if you do start taking an over-the-counter magnesium supplement research the company so you know you are getting real magnesium and take it at night as it will help you sleep naturally.

You may also want to try to change your diet to see if it helps. Some people have a gluten sensitivity that can cause headaches and once eliminated have found relief. And some processed meats like hot dogs, bacon, and other cured meats contain nitrates and nitrites that can cause headaches. Salt, caffeine, MSG, and alcohol can also cause some people headaches. Also, did you know that aged chesses like blue cheese, feta, and Parmesan cheese contain a chemical called tyramine that can cause headaches.

A go-to relaxer I always suggest is a Detox Bath

2 cups apple cider vinegar
1 cup Epsom salt
a few drops lavender oil

Lavender oil is very calming, while Epsom salt is natural magnesium, and my favorite apple cider vinegar helps draw out the uric acid in your body and helps relieve headaches, among a lot of other health benefits I have also previously explained on Apple Cider Vinegar section.

I know I have mentioned what I did, but I will highly suggest if these headaches persist, find a good chiropractor. And if you have a desk job, your body can start having tension headaches, make sure to move and stretch every 20–30 minutes. This is where yoga can be very beneficial.

Now these are not all remedies but these are my go-tos.

The best way to figure out what is causing you pain is to keep a headache journal and document everything throughout your day when you have experienced headaches or migraines to find a pattern.

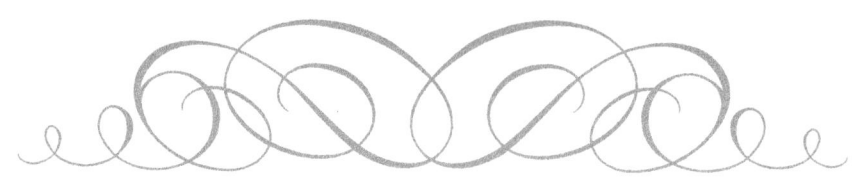

Fevers

Bless the *Lord*, O my soul;
and all my being, bless *His* holy name.
Bless the *Lord*, O my soul,
and forget not all *His* benefits;
He pardons all your iniquities,
He heals all your ills.
He redeems your life from destruction,
He crowns you with kindness and compassion,
He fills your lifetime with good;
Your *Faith* is renewed like the eagle's.

—Psalms 103:1–5

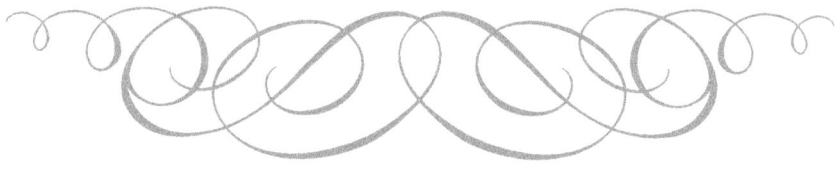

LIVE NATURALLY

There is nothing worse than seeing your loved one sick and feeling helpless that you can't fix it.

My daughter had asthma as a child and would wake unable to breath, we would try steam rooms that seemed to take forever to heat up and try to remain as calm as possible so she didn't get scared and get worse. Many a night I would wrap her up in her blanket and pace outside in front of our house praying for her breathing to restore to normal. She would always cuddle in my arms, trust with her whole heart and God would answer my prayers and her breathing would restore to normal on those very brisk nights.

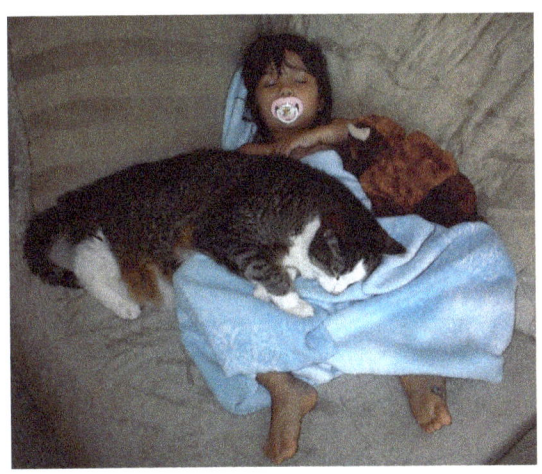

We have also had our fair share of fevers, which are scary too. Although they shouldn't be, fevers are the body's natural way of fighting an infection or a virus. Reducing the fever may actually let the illness last longer.

When using medications to reduce fevers, the body sees them as foreign and needs to now filter the medication, which takes energy that the body could be using to fight the actual problem. Reducing a fever too quickly is not good for the body, you need to do it at a slow rate.

Whenever a fever rears its ugly head you need to keep hydrated, you do not want to risk dehydration and you need to help the body flush out the illness. Lots of water or herbal teas, herbs like ginger, cinnamon, cloves, or peppermint are known as stimulating herbs, when you have a fever, you may feel chilled or unable to get warm, these herbs can help the body heat up, open up your pores and allow your body to sweat which is your body's natural way to cool down and keep a fever from getting too high, it also helps release toxins from the body. Sweating is the body's natural cleaning method, using herbal teas help the body heal itself from what is making you sick.

The teas I tend to are chamomile, elderflower, yarrow, ginger, and peppermint. If you cannot find them in tea bag form you can buy the herbs individually. You can use any of these herbs to make a tea by using loose leaf tea.

Loose Leaf Tea

2 tbsp. of the dried plant
2 cups boiling water

Steep for 10–15 minutes and strain. Sweeten with honey if desired, which is also an amazing tool to use when sick, as it is known to fight infections and heal digestive problems.

It is completely safe to drink 1–2 cups of herbal tea every few hours to help the body when an illness is present.

You also need to support your immune system with probiotics, if you heal the gut you can heal everything. This is where my Kefir Smoothie works very well. I have many reasons why I like this smoothie when my family is not feeling well.

But when it comes to fevers there have been studies that have shown that when a fever develops it pulls calcium from the bones and draws it into the blood where it can be useful to fight infections. This may be why when people have fevers, aches and pains accompany it. So we need to replace that calcium, this kefir smoothie can help and with it being high in antioxidant berries, I always use it as my go-to. Along with a good bone broth soup—grandma was always right with the idea of chicken soup when you're sick!

If your loved one is up for it, a warm bath not cold, will help as well.

Fever Bath

1 cup Epsom Salt
1 tsp. ginger
1 cup apple cider vinegar

It will help alleviate the aches and pains, and will help relax the body. Once a loved one is lying down and comfortable, I always rub a few drops of lavender oil on their feet to help soothe and calm their body and give a few cold cloths for either the forehead, stomach, or feet and let them rest. Rest and sleep is what the body needs so it can do its job and repair itself.

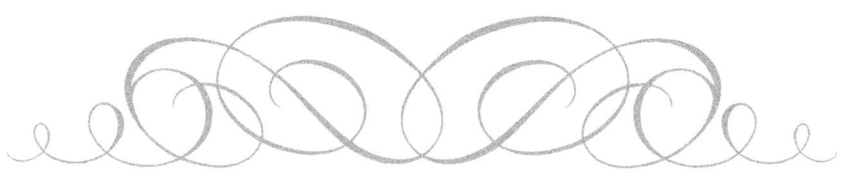

What About Our Girl

Do to *Others*, as you would have them do to *You*.

—Luke 6:31

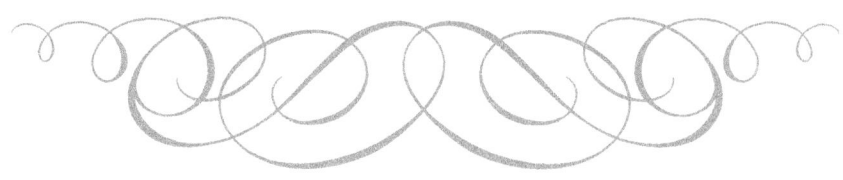

Our girl is better than all of us when it comes to nutrition. Why? Well, she has no choice, she eats what we feed her, but even though this is true she still has a mind of her own and hesitates with new treats or the occasional drop to the floor.

This past lent, a French fry from a fish fry was dropped right in her reach, she smelled it and looked at me like "please tell me you don't eat these!" She wouldn't touch it and had a look of disgust. It really put us all in check!

Our dog is a Shar-Pei and they are known for having a lot of allergies. Our first dog was a Shar-Pei so we knew right away what type of dog food to look for. No grains, no fillers, no corn, and no soy. That wasn't a problem but she still would get the occasional ear infections and throw up randomly. Yes, I should probably step up my game and make her dinners like I make ours.

So our next step's healing the gut, you heal the gut, you heal the ears, and so raw goat's milk it is, every day. I now call her our cat because she loves it so! She has never had another ear infection and it really reduced her bouts of throwing up.

We don't buy dog treats, there are too many ingredients in them that she will have an issue with so fruits and vegetables it is. But an ongoing conversation in our house is what fruits and vegetables can she have and what ones are toxic for dogs.

I think it is time we have a place to reference to, no more questioning.

So here is the first list—what fruits are good for dogs:

- Apples – with the skin are a great source of vitamins A and C, and fiber. Apples can improve digestion and keep away dangerous bacteria in the intestine.

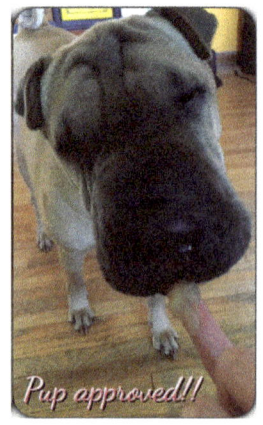

Pup approved!!

If your furry friend does not like apples, try my Applesauce recipe my pup loves it!

- Bananas – are high in vitamins, potassium, biotin, fiber, and copper. But they are also high in sugar and should be given only as a treat. Our girl loves a frozen slice here and there!

- Blueberries – are a super food full of antioxidants, which prevent cell damage in humans and canines. They are also packed with fiber and phytochemicals. If you are trying to teach your dog to catch treats try blueberries!

- Cantaloupe – contains vitamins A, B6, and C, beta-carotene, fiber, folate, niacin, and potassium. Cantaloupes promote good eyesight and beta-carotene and vitamin C have been found to reduce the risk of cancer and prevent oxygen damage to cells. Cantaloupe is found to be non-allergenic so this becomes a good fruit to start with your dog if you have never served her or him fruits before.

- Mango – what a great fruit, it is loaded with vitamins A, B6, C, and E but also has potassium and both beta-carotene and alpha-carotene. Always remember, with these fruits, to remove the pits as they contain trace amounts of cyanide and are toxic to dogs.

- Orange – yes! A small dog can have up to 1/3 of a full size orange and a large dog can have a whole orange. Just make sure to peel it and deseed it. Oranges are a rich source of vitamin C, folate, thiamin, potassium, calcium, and magnesium. Oranges also protect against cancer and can ward off viral infections.

- Peaches – cut up fresh peaches are a great source of fiber and vitamin A. They can help fight infections. Discard the pit safely, as with mangoes and pears, the pit contains cyanide, you do not want your dog potentially getting a hold of it.

- Pears – are a great snack high in vitamins C and K, copper, and fiber. The fiber in pears promotes colon health and can be good for dogs that suffer from constipation or irregularity. Just be sure to cut it in small bite-size pieces and remove the core and seeds, as with peaches, these seeds contain trace amounts of cyanide and are toxic to dogs.

- Pineapple – a few pieces of pineapple are a great sweet treat for your dog. Just make sure the prickly outside is removed first. Pineapples are full of vitamins, minerals, and fiber. They also contain bromelain, which is an enzyme that helps dogs absorb proteins much easier.

- Pumpkin – is rich in vitamins A and C, and beta-carotene another good thing for our pooches eyes. Pumpkins are high in fiber, potassium, zinc, calcium, and magnesium. Pumpkin is also helpful in intestinal health. If your dog experiences diarrhea or constipation, try a few teaspoons of pumpkin.

- Raspberries – are fine in moderation. They are high in fiber, antioxidants, manganese, and vitamin C. They are especially good for senior dogs as they have anti-inflammatory properties, which can take the pain and pressure off the joints. But limit your serving because they do contain slight amounts of the toxin xylitol, which can cause low blood sugar. That being said, your dog would have to eat multiple cups of raspberries. To be safe, stay under a cup of raspberries for a large dog, myself, I only give her 2 or 3 raspberries for a treat.

- Strawberries – they are high in sugar so you should only offer them occasionally for a treat but they are full of fiber and vitamin C. Strawberries contain an enzyme that can help whiten your dog's teeth as she or he eats them!

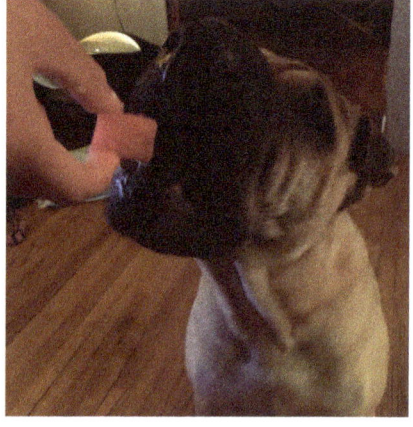

- Watermelon – yay! Our favorite! Watermelon is made of 92% water and is excellent for hydration and the skin. It is a good source of vitamins A, B6, and C, dietary fiber, potassium, and magnesium. Make sure your watermelon is either seedless or you remove the seeds before offering to your four-legged friend.

- Zucchini and squashes – are good sources of vitamins A, C, and some B vitamins, potassium, magnesium, and fiber. Zucchini can be anti-inflammatory and can support a healthy coat and skin. It also contains the phytonutrients lutein and zeaxanthin, which are associated with healthy eyes. Even though we think of zucchini and squashes as vegetables, they are actually fruits because they come from a flower.

Now that we talked about fruits, I think it is time to talk about vegetables and which ones our furry little dog friends can have.

- Bell peppers (all colors) – are a great source of vitamins A, C, E, K, and several B vitamins. They are also rich in beta-carotene, which can prevent cancer and decrease the chances of cataracts, other eye ailments, and arthritis in aging dogs.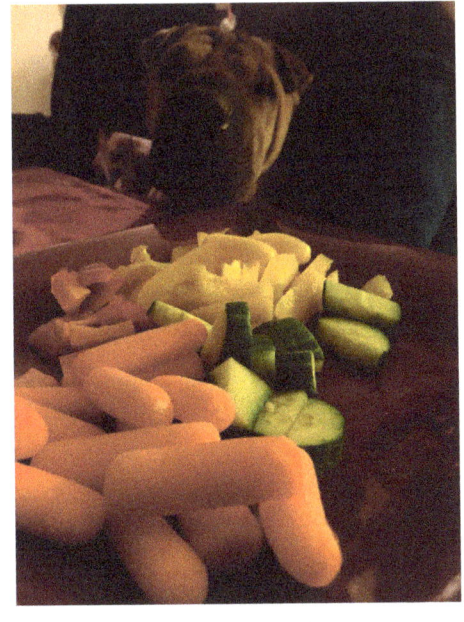

- Bok choy – is good for healthy, strong bones and teeth. It is also good for the heart while protecting against cancer. Bok choy is packed with Vitamins A, C, and K, calcium, and potassium.

- Carrots – this is one of our favorites and it is very good to know they have the same benefits for dogs as they do humans. Carrots have high levels of beta-carotene, which are great for the eyes, as we know. They are also high in fiber and are loaded with vitamins A, C, and K. They also help clean the teeth and gums—a natural toothbrush!

- Celery – improves heart health and can lower blood pressure while helping to fight cancer. Celery is rich in vitamins A, B, and C, calcium, potassium, phosphorus, iron, and sodium. Celery is known to reduce nervousness in animals and acts as an acid neutralizer. Celery also freshens your dog's breath!

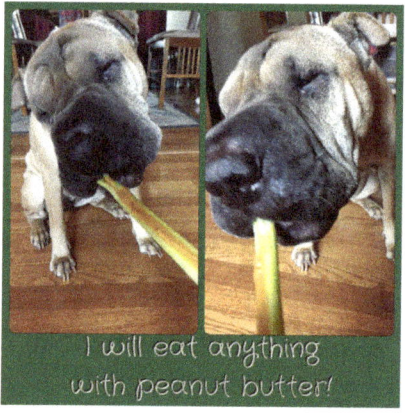

I will eat anything with peanut butter!

- Cucumbers – are loaded with vitamins B, C, and K as well as potassium, copper, magnesium, and biotin. Another favorite of our girls!

- Green beans – are high in vitamins A, C, and K, fiber, calcium, copper, folic acid, iron, niacin, manganese, potassium, riboflavin, thiamin, and beta-carotene. They also contain omega 3 fatty acids, which contribute to cardiovascular benefits and they help promote bone health.

- Green peas – specifically snow peas, sugar snap peas, and garden or English peas. Fresh never canned. Peas are among the healthiest human snack for dogs, they are a great source of vitamins A, K, and the B vitamins. They are also packed with minerals like iron, potassium, zinc, and magnesium, rich in protein and high in fiber. Peas also contain lutein, an antioxidant good for the eyes, skin, and the heart. And as far as the pod goes, if a human can eat it, so can your dog, but a garden pea must be shelled and don't eat that pod. Be cautious with pods, they can get caught in your dog's throat leading to choking. Always remember, dogs do not chew as much as we do.

- Potatoes – contain lots of iron, but never serve them raw or mashed. Make sure they are washed, peeled, and either boiled or baked. When giving them to your dog, cut them in bite-sized pieces and make sure they are cooled.

- Spinach – this nutrient-dense green has twice as much iron as other greens. It is a good source of fiber, calcium, potassium, vitamins A, B6, and K. Spinach can ward off inflammatory and cardiovascular problems as well as cancer.

- Sweet potatoes – are heart healthy, easy on the digestive track, and contribute in lowering blood pressure. They are high in fiber, beta-carotene, vitamins A, C, E, and B vitamins. Serve in bite-size pieces and make sure they are cooked, never give your dog a raw potato.

It may seem weird that there is a maybe list, but there is because some of these are perfectly safe as long as you are using caution and feeding your dog the parts that are safe. I would like to think that all animal lovers treat their animals the way they would like to be treated and therefore, if they are feeding their animals the healthiest foods available to help them live a long loving life then they will make sure to be cautious with these fruits and vegetables.

- Apricots – like cherries, the seeds, leaves, and stems are toxic to dogs. The pulps of the fruit dogs are able to eat. You need to be very cautious that your dog does not have access to any other part of the plant. They also contain cyanide and can result in respiratory failure and death.

- Broccoli – is safe but in small quantities. Looking at broccoli you would think, what could be wrong? But broccoli contains a potentially harmful ingredient called isothiocyanates, which can cause mild to potentially severe gastric irritation in some dogs.

Broccoli stalks have been known to cause obstruction in the esophagus of some dogs. Broccoli is high in fiber and vitamin C.

- Cherries – the fleshy part around the seed is fine, it's the cherry plant and seeds that contain cyanide and are toxic to dogs. Cyanide disrupts the cellular oxygen transport, which means that your dog's blood cells can't get enough oxygen. If your dog eats cherries, be on the lookout for dilated pupils, difficulty in breathing, and red gums. These may be signs of cyanide poisoning.

- Tomato plants – while the actual tomato is very beneficial to dogs, the plant itself is quite toxic. The stems, leaves and unripened fruit can cause gastrointestinal upset. While they may need to consume quite a bit of the plant to be dangerous, it is best to keep these plants out of reach of our furry friends.

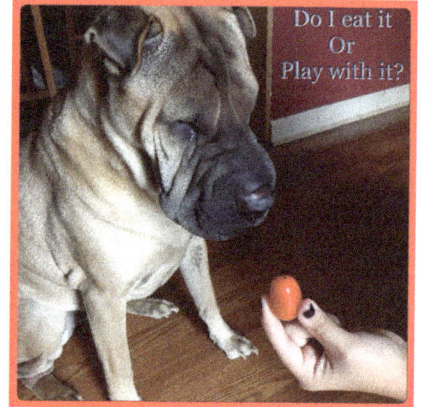

Now for the list every dog owner needs to know—the fruits and vegetables that are toxic to our fur babies. This list is not something to play with, just stay away from them and keep them out of reach!

- Apple seeds – are just like the pits of the cherries and they are highly toxic because they contain cyanide. Because these seeds are smaller, your dog may need to eat a few apples to suffer toxicity. Better safe than sorry, keep apples out of reach of your furry friend. I keep mine in the

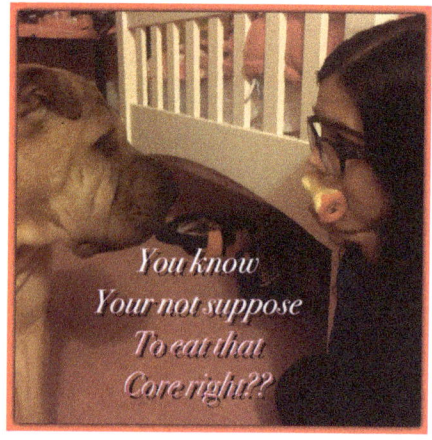

refrigerator and when sharing, I cut them in bite-size pieces and discard the whole core.

- Asparagus – is not unsafe for your dog to eat but are too tough and could cause a choking hazard. If you cook them down to soften you will lose all nutritional benefits. Go for something else that will actually benefit your dog.

- Chives, garlic, leeks and onions – onions are considered more aggressive in their effects. They can cause your dog's red blood cells to rupture, and can cause vomiting, diarrhea, stomach pain, nausea, lethargy, elevated heart, and respiratory rates, pale gums, and even collapse. I think you would agree, let's keep these veggies just for us humans.

- Currants – carry the same level of toxicity as grapes and raisins. Even if you don't notice sudden vomiting and diarrhea after your dog eats currants, take your dog to the vet, currants can cause severe renal failure.

- Grapes and raisins – my first fur baby loved grapes, she would hold it between her paws and suck the middle out before she ate the skin. Well, she definitely was the exception. Since I learned they could be toxic, our girl now has never had one. It is not worth the risk to find out if she is like her sister (not really, but in our family, she is). Consuming grapes or raisins can lead to irreversible kidney damage. It is best to keep these away from your four-legged friend.

- Green peas – any human food can have its drawbacks, even though the green pea family is very good, as we have mentioned, it will not be good if your fur baby has kidney problems. Peas contain purines, a naturally occurring chemical compound found in some foods and drinks. Purines contain uric acid that is filtered through the kidneys. Too much uric acid can lead to kidney stones and kidney conditions.

- Mushrooms – not all mushrooms are toxic but if you're unable to identify a mushroom species, take your dog to the vet immediately, mushroom toxicity is known to be fatal resulting from seizures, tremors, and organ failure.

- Potatoes (not ripe, green, raw) – you may be surprised since potatoes are in a lot of dry dog foods. But not ripe, green, and raw potatoes are toxic not only to dogs but humans as well. Symptoms include nausea, vomiting, seizures, and heart irregularity.

- Rhubarb – the leaves and stems of rhubarb depletes the calcium levels in our dogs' bodies, this can result in renal failure and other medical problems.

Now we all know that dogs don't chew like we do, so make sure to give little portions, depending on the food, offer raw or slightly steamed. Deseed everything! And if steaming never add any seasonings or oils. When serving any leafy greens, if your dog is like mine, she or he may not eat them raw, so cut in slices and steam a few minutes. After you have cooked them cool completely and rough chop them and separate them before feeding so they don't gobble them down. These lists I am sure do not include everything but it starts as a good guide. I have done my research and encourage you to do the same, if you question something you can give your fur baby that I didn't include, look into it and then let me know, I always want to learn more too!

Now in telling you all of these, it is important, I state, that dogs do not need fruits and vegetables in their diets the way humans do. They are carnivorous in the wild and only eat vegetation when meat sources are scarce. So, as an occasional snack or treat is perfectly safe. And your dog will love that she or he gets to enjoy what you enjoy!

And now another tip with my favorite apple cider vinegar! Add a teaspoon to a quart of drinking water for every 40 pounds for your fur baby to keep the fleas away, it also will help improve your dog's skin from the inside out!

Let's keep our companions healthy and safe!

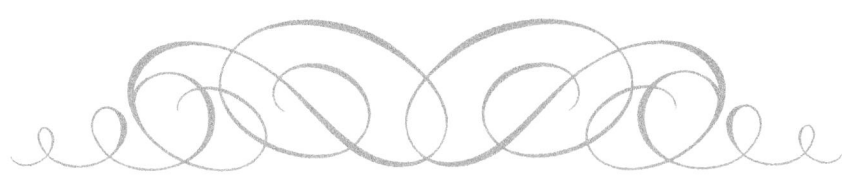

Where Are We Going

Even to your old age *I* am the same, even when your hair is grey *I* will *bear* you; it is *I* who have done this, *I* who will continue, and *I* who will *carry* you to safety.

—Isaiah 46:4

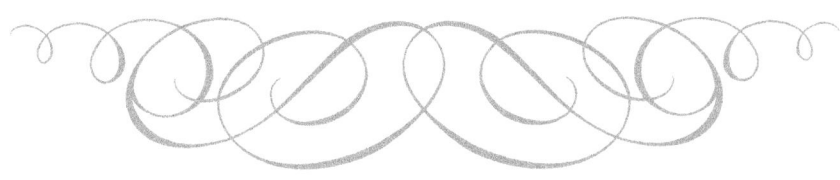

During this journey of writing this, yes, now I can call it a book! I have done a lot of different things. It has taken a lot of soul searching because I do not like talking about my health and why I believe in the things I do. Writing this book has completely taken me out of my comfort zone. I have had to relive the past and how I got through the things I did. I have had to really put all my beliefs, techniques, and knowledge I have learned on paper, which seems easy but sometimes is the hardest part. I have had to make every single recipe I have shared with you, photograph every recipe, and do something I never do—measure ingredients! My family and friends are not complaining, they have gotten very good meals this past year.

During the time I have been writing, typing, and creating it had become the Lenten season.

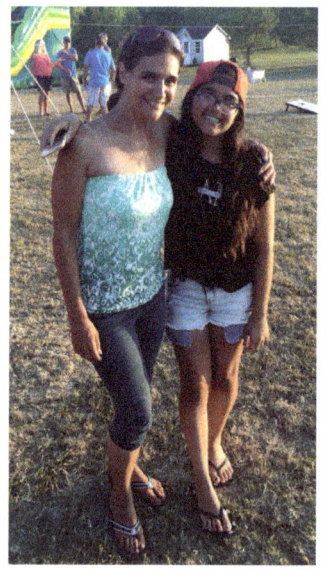

It is no secret of my deep religious beliefs. Now Lent to me, as a child, was always giving up something you enjoy. But in my adult years it became more about spreading love, peace, and not judging others. Not letting the negative consume you, only allowing the mind to be positive.

You know, something we should practice and do every day. Sounds easy, but for some reason, it's not and it is something that if done, can be spread onto others and hopefully make a more peaceful world.

Well, during this Lenten season, I decided to jump all in spiritually and nutritionally. So, not only everything I just explained but also more prayer, meditation, expressing my thoughts on paper, truly listening to God through all the signs he shares with us constantly and we just need to be open to listen. And yes, giving some things up, so while I have been creating all of these meals for my family and friends, I have had to really restrain from my own temptations. So, what did I give up? I gave up bread, sugars, and alcohol of any kind. Yes, all at once, now this is a bit drastic but for me it needed to happen like this. I am not big on sweets so that one has always been an easy one, but breads, pizza, and pasta now, that was a hard one. I didn't think I could do it but I did! And I have continued on that path, which has been the best feeling!

I have learned a lot about temptation, some would say the devil knocking at your door, I'm not sure, all I know is when you decide to do something, there will always be something trying to change your mind or get in your way. I used to call them walls, but now I think it's the universe trying to make you stronger and prove to you, you can do anything you put your mind to. It is not easy to not give in or give up when things are trying to tear you down. But somehow you have to dig deep inside yourself and know where your core beliefs lay and not be afraid to live the life you see fit, you were created for a path of your own, not someone else's, so it is very important to not let anything stand in your way no matter how hard it is to continue down the path you feel you are destined to create.

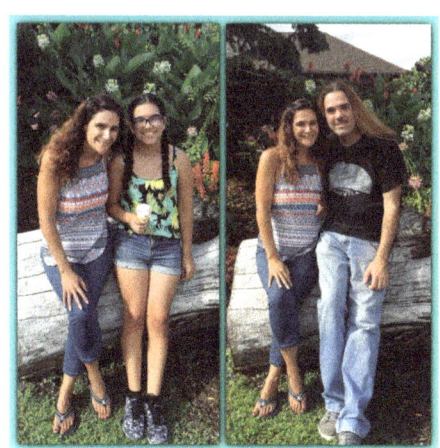

So I pose the question to myself—where are we going?

Well, that's a tough one, does anyone truly know for sure what the future has in store for us? But I do know I am not stopping, my creative mind is ever turning and I will continue to make products and recipes and share them with anyone that is interested.

These past few months, I have put my mind to many things and I get a bit rattled with all the information in my head. It may still be effects from the head injury, but I refuse to look at it as a negative.

During this time, not only have I been doing all this work for what has become my book, but also have expanded my skincare line and seem to be creating all the time. I started making our own products just for our family's use, then it became for our friends and extended family when they were unable to use some products on the market. It is becoming much bigger than my little circle and needs to be shared with everyone on a similar path as myself, wanting to live a purer life with as little chemicals and additives as possible, a healthier way of living.

Going forward, I will continually treat my body with the respect that it was created for, that to me means making sure to feed it the best way I can. I eat cleaner than most people I know and still know there is room to make better choices and not feel that I am ever abstaining from anything. I will continue to inform the people that want to know, and will never pass judgment on others or push my beliefs.

It is funny, the things I do I truly don't push onto my family, but they watch and it is true what they say about your children becoming a form of yourself in different ways. In the past few weeks my daughter told me how proud she was of herself, of staying conscience of her water intake and how many glasses she has had at school and at home. She explained how much better her body has felt, she does watch me and yes, I comment when she has softball games to stay hydrated, but most of what I teach is by what I do without words. She also is getting older on me and now out with friends when I am not around, I only pray that her choices stay good. And I know they will, she jokes that her friends always comment on her healthier lunches and she explains to them how good they are while they eat their very unhealthy school lunches.

During exam week, they decided to order a pizza, as you know, we make our own. She didn't want to be rude so she ate a slice and came home pretty sick to her stomach and told me, "Mom, it was so greasy and gross but I didn't want to be rude and not eat. But next time I will pass." It did not taste good and made her feel awful. Sometimes we need to learn about food the hard way, we all have done it. And when you start eating cleaner you will notice some foods that never bothered you in the past may bother you now, because you have created a cleaner environment for your body.

Sundays have always been our family day, and we end our night with God and go to our church. In the summer we take family walks to and from church. This summer, my daughter's friend was going to be moving out of state, all the kids tended to hang out more and more each week, which was so nice to see even though you knew it would come to an end. One Sunday, they wanted to come back to our house for a fire in the yard, my daughter explained to them that we go to church on Sunday nights and they said they would come. Never hold back on your beliefs, never push them either, but you may be surprised that others may want to do exactly what you are and talk to God on a Sunday night too. I am so grateful that I have raised my daughter to never feel she has to change her ways or her beliefs for others, and she has an amazing group of friends. Love watching these kids grow into mini-adults!

It has always been hard for me to not worry about what others think, but by doing that I have not created the path I was put on this earth for. I have always put others' needs before my own, and will continue to do that because that is my nature. But now, when I publish this book, I will not think twice if someone doesn't like it or what I have to say, in reality, I truly needed to create this project so I could get my thoughts out of my head and on paper, somewhere concrete that I could refer too—in one place! Something I could pass on to my daughter, although the cutest person she is, she told me she wants to keep my old writings because that is where it all began and what she has watched me do throughout the years. When she said that, it blessed my heart in such a way! But there goes my idea of trying to minimize papers. Ha ha.

I hope you liked my book and learned a thing or two, I would love to hear if you made any of my recipes and how you liked them. Send me a message, I would love to hear from you!

And I will close with the best advice I have been given during this journey, from my loving daughter, "You be you, and don't worry about anything else."

Have a blessed day!

Love,

Andréa

Index

Flax Egg 32

Breakfast

Andrea's Easy on the Go 41
Cinnamon Roll 41
Healthy Fat Shake 42
Monkey Heaven 42
Thin Mintalicious 43
Berry-Licious 43
Nuts About Berries 43
Banana Milkshake 44
Banana Nut Shake 44
Café Latte 45
Iced Mocha 45
Neapolitan 46
Vanilla Chai 46
Avocado Toast 47
Broccoli Cheese Eggs or Egg Muffins 48
Cheesy Hash Brown Casserole 49
Healthier Hash Brown Bake 50
Home Fries 51
My Homemade Pancake Mix 52
Blueberry Pancakes 52
Chocolate Chip Pancakes 53
Gluten-Free Buckwheat Kefir Pancakes 54
Yogurt Parfait 55

Soups

Momma's Broccoli Soup 58
Momma's Chili 59
Cream of Broccoli Cauliflower Soup 60
Creamy Butternut Squash Soup with Quinoa 61
Lentil, Kale, and Potato Soup 62
Potato Leek Soup 63
Smoked Turkey Soup 64
Tomato Basil Soup 65
Momma's Organic Vegetable Soup 66

Salads

Avocado Salad 70
Avocado, Artichoke Chopped Salad 71
Beet Avocado Salad 72
Buffalo Chicken Salad 73
Brussels Sprout Slaw 74
Guac Lentil Salad 75
Hummus Salad 76
Kohlrabi Salad 77
Lemon, Garbanzo, Tuna Salad 78
Potato Salad 79
Tuna Noodle Salad 80
Vegetable Pasta Salad 81
Watermelon Salad 82

Sides

Baked Beans 85
Buffalo Cauliflower 86
Easy Buffalo Cauliflower 87
Garlic Kale 88
Mashed Potatoes 89
Mashed Sweet Potatoes with Cheddar 90

Roasted Asparagus 91
Roasted Asparagus with Garlic 91
Roasted Beets 92
Steamed Beets 92
Roasted Broccoli...93
Roasted Cauliflower 94
Roasted Spaghetti Squash 95
Scalloped Potatoes 96
Stuffing 97
Zucchini Marinara 98

Sandwiches

Avocado Vegetable Panini... 102
Black Bean Burger... 103
Buffalo Chicken Salad Wrap.. 104
Hummus Wrap 105
Quinoa Cake.. 106
Ranch Chicken Salad Panini 107
Salmon Burger 108
Tuna Artichoke Melt 109
Tuna Burger 110
Tuna Salad Sandwich with Pickles 111
Turkey Apple Panini.. 112

Meals

Broccoli Quinoa Bake 115
Cauliflower Alfredo 116
Cauliflower Fried Rice.. 117
Cauliflower Pizza Crust 118
Chicken Asparagus Bake 119
Chicken Cacciatore 120
Chicken Souvlaki 121
Spinach Artichoke Falafel 122

Farro 123
Lazy Lasagna Bake 124
Lazy Pierogi 125
Loaded Sweet Potato 126
Pierogi 127
Salsa Quinoa Bake 128
Spinach and Squash Mini Manicotti 129
Squash Mac and Cheese 130
Vegetable Lasagna 131

Condiments

Avocado Hummus 134
Beet Hummus 135
Garlic Hummus 136
Greek Dressing 137
Guacamole 138
Momma's Sauce 139
Pesto 140
Pickles 141
Red Pepper Hummus 142
Ricotta Cheese Mixture 143
Salsa 144
Vinaigrette 145

Party Time

Buffalo Wing Dip 148
Buffalo Wing Pizza 149
Pesto Pizza 150
Rosabella Pizza 151
Spinach Artichoke Avocado Dip 152
Spinach Artichoke Dip 153
Stuffed Peppers 154
Swiss Chard Pizza 155

Vegetable Pizza 156
White Pizza 157
Zakuska 158

Desserts
Apple Crisp 161
Apple Sauce 162
Beet Brownies 163
Caramel Apple Nachos 164
Cheesecake Bites 165
Chocolate Chick Bars 166
Cinnamon Sugar Almonds 167
Cinnamon Tortillas 168
Cookie Dough Balls 169
Fruit Salsa 170
Hot Fudge 171
Ice Cream 172
Ice Cream Cakes 173
Pumpkin Dip 174
Rhubarb Bread 175
Spicy Almonds 176
Strawberry Rhubarb Crumble 177
Watermelon Cake 178
Whip Cream 179

Home Remedies
Kefir Smoothie 40
My ACV Water 195
Detox Bath 203
Loose Leaf Tea 207
Fever Bath 208

About the Author

Andréa is a mom to a beautiful girl and a special education teacher aide. She started her career in business and accounting, after having her daughter she realized her life had changed and needed to be home with her family more and find a different path in life. She has always had a passion for photography and has been known to photograph weddings and musicians throughout the years.

Andréa has been on her wellness journey since her teen years. She has always researched and experimented theories on herself to stay as healthy and natural as possible. She loves to cook and has found a niche in making not-so-good-for-you food actually be good-for-you with the right kind of ingredients.

As many nowadays, she has had health problems but has always chosen to stay as natural as possible and trust in the Lord that it is part of the bigger plan. Throughout her journey she has created her own skincare line, continuing in her beliefs of using what God has given us.

CPSIA information can be obtained
at www.ICGtesting.com
Printed in the USA
BVHW02s1652250918
528079BV00017B/26/P